I'M HUNGRY! I'M BORED!

Eat and Play Your Way to Better Health, a Leaner Physique, and a Happier Life!

For Adults and Tots through Teens

Carol McCormick

American Council on Exercise
Certified Personal Trainer
Certified Health Coach

www.carolmccormick.com

Celestial Press
New York

The author is a certified personal trainer and a certified health coach through the American Council on Exercise. And even though ACE is internationally recognized as one of the top fitness organizations in the world, neither she nor they are qualified to dispense medical advice. Therefore, this book is not a substitute for the professional medical advice, diagnosis or treatment of a physician or a registered dietitian. Readers should consult appropriate healthcare professionals for the diagnosis and treatment of any medical or health conditions and before participating in strenuous activities.

The safety and well-being of children is of utmost importance while participating in all physical activities mentioned in this book. Therefore, all activities that have the potential to incur bodily harm should be performed with proper headgear, footwear, kneepads, sunscreen, and other precautionary measures to minimize or prevent injuries. All suggested activities should be done in a safe environment, and young children should always be under adult supervision.

The health and nutrition information contained in this book is widely available and easily verifiable on many government health websites. Links to these sites and additional resources are provided at the end of this book.

To the joy of my heart, Gavin Estep

Books by Carol McCormick

Talk to Me! Listen to Me!
Keys to Improve Communication and
Questions to Deepen Relationships

The Missing Piece
Award-winning Inspirational Love Story

Your Special Gift
A Preteen Primer to the Facts of Life

Window Pains
Modeling Positive Behaviors

TABLE OF CONTENTS

I'M HUNGRY!

I'M BORED!

I'M HUNGRY!

PRE-GAME WARM-UP

"I'm Hungry! I'm Bored!" How many times have you heard these words from your children? Those who are old enough to take care of themselves usually do so by raiding the fridge or ransacking the cupboards, or by flopping down in front of a PC, TV or other electronic device for hours. If your children are young, you have more of a say in their eating habits and their time spent with the one-eyed-cyber-monsters. Older kids, now that's a different story. The task becomes a tug-of-war, because teens don't always listen or want to do what's best for them. Not only that, but there's the added challenge of competing with their friends who may sway them from your good intentions and influence.

Well come a little closer. I've got good news for you. *I'm Hungry! I'm Bored!* can help you and your children make better food choices and encourage positive behaviors by making meaningful activities and good nutrition enjoyable, fun, and exciting. This book will arm you with hundreds of ideas that can help your child thrive in life. Because a child left to himself, when it comes to food, activity, and entertainment, will often take the path of least resistance and choose junk food to eat, or the internet to occupy his time, often because he or she doesn't know what else to do. The children who do know their options will still need additional ideas, examples, and encouragement to hoof the higher path on the oftentimes bumpy road of life.

That being said, I present to you a virtual goldmine of goodies. You hold in your hands, hundreds of hours of gathered facts from credible sources, along with a few gems of my own, condensed and funneled into one treasure chest for easy reading and access.

I've done the footwork for you and provided the *what, why*, and *how-to* of nutrition and weight loss by defining the problems, offering solutions, and then presenting guidelines to carry them through. The *I'm Bored!* section offers hundreds of links and suggestions to great books, movies, places to go, things to do, questions to ask, jobs to perform, and services to volunteer, all-of-which help develop the intellect, confidence, and feelings of fulfillment. Many of these ideas may also deter the hand-to-mouth eating habit that often accompanies boredom.

Some of this info may be new to you, while other parts may be a reminder of things you already know, or knew, but may have forgotten from your childhood. If that is the case, think of this info as a gentle press of the recall button, a prompt to use as a tool in shaping the course of your child's life.

The suggestions are geared for children three years-old up to the age of about eighteen, but everything in this book will also work for adults too, aside from a few of the activity ideas. But hey, who knows, you may enjoy them too!

I often use the second person pronoun, *you*, in this book when I am speaking about your child, but since you, the parent, guardian, or caregiver, are the ones reading this information, buying the products, preparing the food, taking them places, or guiding them in other ways, I'm really speaking to all of *you*, so you can inform and help them.

I also encourage you to lead by example in this new adventure. If you spend a lot of time in front of a television or computer screen, your kids will be more inclined to do so too. If you exercise and have many interests and participate in meaningful activities, the odds are in your favor that they will follow suit. If you want your children to eat better, become more active, and to use their time more wisely, you must model these behaviors, because they often don't know any better. Even if they do, they don't have the means to make significant changes, since you're in control of the food that comes into the house, how it's prepared, and whether you order-in or eat-out. You're also in control of their extended recreation, especially if it involves money.

Therefore, you have the power to help them make changes. This whole shebang is a joint effort with you leading the pack. When you make good nutrition, exercise and physical activity a lifestyle, a given, a normal way of living, it becomes a fun and exciting adventure rather than a burden to be endured.

Most of the charts in this book are applicable for adults, if you use the numbers for an eighteen year old, although after 50+ years most of the numbers decline. What you weighed at age eighteen, if a healthy weight, should be maintained throughout your life, with the exception of during a pregnancy. Many people believe that it's normal or even expected to gain weight as they age. The metabolism does slow down with each passing decade, but the major cause of weight gain is simply poor lifestyle choices. If you believe it's a natural occurrence that cannot be avoided, you'll be more inclined to put on the pounds. But if you believe that you can maintain a healthy weight throughout your entire life, or if you believe that you can lose the weight you've gained, you stand a greater chance of seeing it happen. The seeds of success grow in the soil of faith.

If your child needs to lose weight, he or she can win this war and be shielded from a host of "adult" ailments such as Type

2 diabetes, heart disease, and high-blood pressure, *once these behaviors are in place.* The majority of children don't suffer from these diseases, although statistics are rising at an alarming rate, indicating that many children are headed in that direction. Some have already arrived. The habits you instill in them now often follow them into adulthood, where many of these ailments may await them, if there is no intervention.

KIDS JUST WANT TO HAVE FUN

My dad was an avid outdoorsman, so I grew up eating venison, rabbit, and fish with side-dishes of veggies and potatoes, in what most people today would consider tiny portions. My parents couldn't afford to buy junk food such as cakes, cookies, and potato chips, although we did have them on occasion. But even then, they were rationed out in small measures like most people did at that time. My sister and I were given a dime a week to buy ten pieces of penny candy at the corner grocery store. I ate my first Big Mac when I was seventeen years-old, because fast-food restaurants weren't around much before that time.

When I was in high school, girls were required to take home economics. I enjoyed most of the class, but the section on nutrition was so boring to me that halfway through the semester, the teacher sent a warning letter home to my parents, informing them that I was failing the class. The nutrition lessons were dry and boring with their statistics and numbers. I viewed vitamins as useless letters tacked onto food like labels. I could neither relate to, nor see the personal benefits associated with healthy eating. I just wanted to have fun, and I found out later that eating junk food was a lot of fun. It wasn't until after I graduated from high school and moved out of the house and had so much fun, I outgrew my clothes three times in the course of two years.

I wore baggy attire to accommodate my growing girth, but then one day, I saw a photo of myself in my lovely pocketed smock and stretchy polyester pants, and it hit me: I was unpleasingly plump. I tried the latest diet crazes and weight loss quackeries all to no avail, so I began to read everything I could about health, nutrition, and fitness. I was sick and tired of feeling sick and tired, and of being overweight and out of shape, so I did something about it. It took me six more years of gaining and losing weight, over and over again, and then later struggling with eating disorders, before I finally figured out how to eat healthy and how to *maintain* a normal weight.

The content of this book is a result of my sweat, tears, and triumph. I weigh today what I weighed back then, my ideal weight at age eighteen. I never feel deprived and I don't deny myself a treat now-and-then, because I know how to play the numbers game to keep the score in my favor. A sweet indulgence *on occasion* also prevents the pendulum effect. You know, that all-or-nothing feast-or-famine insanity cycle? I stay on track by using the ideas that you are about to read. The same track I've trod with little fluctuation for over thirty years.

Kids are all about having fun or doing things they enjoy. The problem is that when you make changes to their diets, they typically feel like you're taking away their fun, and then often rebel. To keep this from happening, you must replace the empty space with something else, because life cannot exist in a vacuum.

To remove one negative "fun" thing, you must replace it with another fun or enjoyable thing that isn't junk food related. As you begin this transition, appeal to their good sense through logic and reasoning. They must see, not the things that they will lose (except weight, if needed), but the things that they will gain instead: delicious whole food that tastes good, to keep them healthy and strong. Foods that promote clearer skin, sharper thinking, and happier feelings of well-being, along with activities that boost energy levels, increase muscle mass, and improve self- confidence. They will also gain knowledge and experience when connected to fun, educational, and interesting activities.

Modifying children's diets and behaviors can be done with the aforementioned perks as incentives, but the motor that drives them in a new direction (in the beginning, until they internalize these behaviors) must ultimately come from your firm guidance. The rewards must outweigh the temporary benefit of eating "fun" junk food, or being inactive and unproductive. As you continue to read, you will discover the tools to chip away unhealthy habits and the blueprints to build new ones.

FROM CRAZY DAZE TO HAPPY DAYS

One of the most amazing cases for the benefits of good nutrition and fitness took place at Appleton Alternative Charter High School in Wisconsin. The establishment began as a sanctuary for children who had a history of skipping school and being disruptive in class. The school was also a place for those who exhibited psychological and emotional problems, and for those who struggled with drug addictions and violent behaviors, and for those who had broken the law in one form or another.

In its early days, the school had no cafeteria so the children drank sodas and ate candy bars, chips, and other junk food from vending machines throughout the day. Teachers noticed that after the students ate these snacks they were bad-tempered and lacked focus. Bouts of anger, swearing, and complaints of feeling ill and tired were also par-for-the-course.

Change came when the school set up an exercise area with weights, treadmills, and stationary bikes. The school also joined forces with Natural Ovens Bakery to open an onsite kitchen and dining area. The school removed the vending machines and replaced them with water coolers, and then began serving nutrient dense whole foods for both breakfast and lunch.

The results were astounding! The staff noticed behavioral improvements almost immediately. The children became calmer. Concentration and attitudes improved, while inappropriate behavior waned. Physical complaints and mid-day hunger also declined. But the most astonishing observation, according to Principal LuAnn Coenen, was that "vandalism, drug and weapons violations, dropout and expulsion rates, and suicide attempts are virtually nonexistent."

To make sure these new behaviors weren't a fluke, the staff tested this program by having a junk food day where the students were given sugar-filled drinks, candy bars, chips and desserts to eat. By the end of the day, the children had reverted back to many of their previous misbehaving. It was as though some force had taken control of their minds, bodies, and emotions, changing their personalities. [1]

Coincidence? I think not. I had experienced many of these same negative feelings and effects for years: The wild rollercoaster of emotions, the crazy behaviors, the all-or-nothing pendulum effect. Not a pretty picture. The Appleton program worked because the school implemented a fitness program and changed their menu to include healthy food, but it also succeeded because it was done in a controlled environment. The children had no choice but to eat nutritious food, for two meals of the day anyway, or else go hungry. Most of us don't have the luxury of someone buying and preparing our meals to keep us on track.

The more choices we have in life, the more difficult it is to choose what's right. In the beginning of my health journey, I had all the facts in my head. I knew what to eat and how to exercise. I did them both quite often too, but something was missing from my regimen. Trying to eat right and exercise regularly was like climbing a mudslide and getting halfway to the top, but then sliding back down again. There were too many sizzling, sweet, or gooey temptations knocking at my door. (It would have helped not to order in.) But then I finally "got it." Instead of heading straight up the summit, I changed my path and took a roundabout way.

One of my greatest discoveries came when I realized that losing weight and gaining physical strength and endurance, by eating right and exercising, should not be my sole focus. I also needed to gain *inner*-strength and endurance by feeding my spirit and mind wholesome thoughts via what I was listening to, watching, and reading. And I needed to exercise my social muscles by reaching out to others and doing things for them, and with them. Instead of delaying my progress up the hill, these new behaviors became the stepping stones that guided me to the peak of the mound. I also found that the more repetitions I did in these areas, the stronger I became in other areas of my life too.

DON'T MAKE FOOD A REWARD OR ENTERTAINMENT

Children are not puppies that need little treats every time they do a good deed or accomplish a small feat. Adults should not use food as bribery to inspire a child to behave. Food should not be a reward for positive behavior, like a prize after winning a game. Food should not be a main source of entertainment such as when going out to eat, when ordering in, or when buying food at the grocery store.

Whew! That was tough to write, because I've done those things myself. A few M&Ms work wonders when potty-training a toddler, yet learning to tinkle on target is not a perpetual event. The problem is that what began as a treat for the child becomes an expectation. What began as an occasional reward becomes the motivator of choice to coax children into good behavior. The ironic part about this is the more treats and sweets they eat, the worse their actions often become when the blood sugar spikes and dips kick in, or when they don't feel good about themselves because they're overweight.

Children are *more* motivated by random rewards, rather than a steady stream of goodies and treats. If a seal in training is fed all the time, the food loses its power to motivate. Trainers know there are other ways to reinforce and reward positive behaviors, such as with eye-contact, tone of voice, praise, and affection. It works with animals. It works with people too.

When a child does something well, and you feel that he or she deserves a treat, replace the food reward with your *time* and *attention*. This can be done by way of appreciation, sincere praise in a loving tone of voice, tender or playful affection, or a small non-food gift or fun activity.

Give them a steady dose of your time and attention by taking a genuine interest in their lives. Participate in a few of the activities suggested in this book. Make a fuss over their accomplishments, no matter how large or small. Give them a hug or a pat on the back, especially when they do something well. Ask a question or make a positive comment about something they've achieved, such as, "Did you do that all by yourself? It's beautiful!" or "You did a great job!" Thank them for favors they do for you, or for jobs that they've done on their own, or for any acts of generosity they've shown to you or others. Praise and appreciation will encourage your children to repeat these positive behaviors.

You may also try buying a few plastic trophies, blue ribbons, or award certificates to acknowledge and reinforce their progress. Maybe he or she is eating healthier, or becoming more active, or showing more kindness to others. All improvement deserves recognition, to encourage the continuation of the positive behavior. Hold a ceremony with as much fanfare as possible, as you celebrate and present him or her with the award. A healthy, home-cooked meal served on a special honorary plate even becomes a tradition much more anticipated and appreciated than a fast food "reward" served in a paper bag.

Stoop down to their level and make direct eye-contact when saying, "I love you," "I've missed you," or "I'm proud of you." Make the statements more potent by using the pronoun *I*. Saying, "Love you" is great most of the time, but it's less direct and powerful. The missing pronoun combined with slang, such as, "Love *ya*," is also fine as a casual term of endearment such as when bidding a person farewell, but saying, "*I* love *you,*" aims straight for the heart and connects the dots to tether their heart to yours.

This is the "food" that nourishes a child and helps him or her thrive in life. Children have an instinctive desire and hunger for love and attention, as we all do. Feeding them boatloads of sugar, salt, and fat is not a loving deed. Emotional nourishment is what a child deeply needs more than sweet-filled treats or high-fat snacks.

When recognition, attention, and quality moments are provided on a regular basis, a child's self-confidence will bloom and his or her spirit will begin to soar. When children are deprived of these innate needs, some may try to fill the void with inferior food, or possibly even alcohol, drugs, or promiscuous sex.

WEIGHT IS JUST A NUMBERS GAME

Childhood obesity is at an all-time high in the United States. Since 1980 the numbers have steadily risen and have almost tripled, so that one in every three children is now categorized as overweight or obese. An alarming 70% of obese teens have either high cholesterol or high blood pressure, both of which are precursors of heart disease. Many are pre-diabetic or already have Type 2 diabetes. Another study on obesity discovered that a staggering two-billion people, *almost one-third of the entire world*, is now overweight or obese. [2]

Losing weight is a numbers game. A simple math equation. Calories consumed must not exceed the calories needed each day or they will be stored as fat. Gaining and losing weight is a matter of math and there's no other way around it. Here is the basic formula to lose weight:

1. Eat FEWER calories than usual each day.
2. Burn MORE calories than usual each day.

For example, if someone cuts 300 calories from his or her diet and burns 300 calories through exercise every day, this 600 calorie a day deficit will force the body to tap into its fat reserves and burn it off as fuel. This calorie slash and burn will result in a person losing just over one pound in a week.

Yikes! That's it? Yes, I know, but it takes 3,500 calories to gain or to lose one pound. This is why it's so important to stay physically active and to *choose foods wisely*, so that every calorie counts toward health.

The good news is the more a child weighs, the faster he or she can lose it. When an overweight person eats the recommended amount of calories, there is a bigger reduction in calories compared to what he or she is accustomed to eating. This makes the weight drop faster.

Another advantage overweight children have is that they will burn more calories as they become more active, because their body weight works on their behalf like "weights" when they participate in any type of strenuous sport.

KEEPING SCORE

You keep score in any sport by measuring your points against your opponent's points. The numbers provide facts to make an evaluation about who won the game. What if I said that the Red Team had 40 points? You may say, "Okay, so what about it?" The number is pointless and means nothing to you, if you have nothing to compare it to.

What if I said that eight Buffalo chicken wings have 588 calories, a can of soda has 136 calories, and a tablespoon of blue cheese dressing has 73 calories, for a grand total of 797 calories? Again, this number means nothing to you if you have nothing to compare it to. But, if I tell you that a 12 year-old girl should limit her food intake to 1,600 calories a day, then you know she's halfway to her daily calorie limit with this one little fatty snack.

Reading labels is like having a game plan and the opponent's playbook. The problem is that reading a label is often like reading Greek. Therefore, the first rule of deciphering a food label is to know *your* numbers (daily requirements and limits), so you can compare them to *their* numbers.

Estimated calorie requirements

AGE AND GENDER	TOTAL DAILY CALORIE NEEDS
Children 2-3	1000
Children 4-8	1200-1400
Girls 9-13	1600
Boys 9-13	1800
Girls 14-18	1800
Boys 14-18	2200
Women 19-30	2000
Men 19-30	2400
Women 31-50	1800
Men 31-50	2200
Women 51+	1600
Men 51+	2000

Figure 1. These numbers apply to those who get less than 30 minutes a day of moderate physical activity *beyond normal daily activities*. Adapted from the USDA Center for Nutrition Policy and Promotion's at ChooseMyPlate.gov.

Once you know your calorie number, it's easy to do a quick calculation when buying or preparing food. The quick assessment idea is similar to estimating your grocery bill when you place items on the conveyor belt before cashing out of the store. When you do this, you may be a dollar or two off, but you have a general idea of what your bill will be, so there are no big surprises when you're ready to pay.

I don't count calories, but I always check and estimate to see if a food contains a lot of them. I glance at the fat numbers on labels and restaurant websites too. This way I know where my boundaries are, so I don't cross them. If the calories or fat numbers are high, I eat a *small portion* of it, or choose a different food. That's it. There's really no need to count calories when eating high fiber foods such as whole grains, veggies, and fruit, or low-fat protein, because they're naturally low in calories and they're also very filling. It's the fake food made in factories and the high-fat food prepared in restaurants that you need to watch.

On this same line of thinking, you should also be aware of how many calories are burned during physical activity. The following chart is an example of a 154 pound teenage boy who is 5' 10" tall, and the number of calories he will burn while doing the following activities.

Moderate Physical Activities	30 minutes
Hiking	185
Yard work	165
Dancing	165
Bicycling (<10 mph)	145
Walking (3 ½ mph)	140
Weight training (light)	110
Stretching	90
Vigorous Physical Activities	**30 minutes**
Running / jogging (5 mph)	295
Bicycling (over 10 mph)	295
Swimming (slow freestyle laps)	295
Aerobics	240
Walking (4 ½ mph)	230
Heavy yard work (chopping wood)	220
Weight lifting (vigorous)	220
Basketball (vigorous)	220

Figure 2. Adapted from the choosemyplate.gov website

As you continue to read, you will find more charts with age-appropriate numbers that apply to you or your child. When you find the correct numbers, write down the daily limits for *calories, sugar, total fat, saturated fat*, and *salt,* as well as the minimum requirements for *fiber* on an index card.

Fill out one card for each child and one for yourself. (Turn back to the calorie chart on the previous page and write down the applicable numbers.) You may want to take a picture of the cards once they are finished, and keep the information in your Smart Phone. You can also make and save a note in your phone to have these facts with you when grocery shopping or eating out. Here are the six areas to write down now:

1. Calories
2. Sugar
3. Total fat
4. Saturated fat
5. Salt
6. Fiber

Once you have done this, refer to your ranges when reading the sections relating to each topic. More importantly, remember or refer to these numbers when you read food labels in the grocery store, in your home, or in restaurants, so you can make a quick assessment before preparing or purchasing food.

Knowing how to read labels will also protect you and your family from deceptive marketing. For example, Skinny Cow® sounds like a healthy treat, doesn't it? How else would the cow on the cover stay so slim? The name and image give the illusion that you too can be a skinny cow or a skinny chick, if you polish off their products. The trim bovine logo is a powerful motivator and selling point.

Most of their products are lower in calories and fat than similar items, but brands are not always consistent across the board. For example, one itty-bitty ounce of Skinny Cow's

Divine-filled Caramel Chocolates contains 7 grams of fat, 4 grams of saturated fat, and almost 4 teaspoons of sugar. The problem with these products and similar brands are that many people don't stop at one ounce, especially when they believe the food is "safe" to eat (low in calories, fat, or sugar), so they end up eating even more.

Another misleading ploy is famous people owning or endorsing products or restaurants. When athletes approve of a specific food, drink, or restaurant, they are often perceived as health-conscious and trustworthy. As a result, many people buy the products, assuming they are good for them, when they're really not. For example, Magic Johnson, Hall of Fame basketball guard, owns a TGIF and promotes a local Starbucks. Peyton Manning, record-setting quarterback, purchased 21 Papa John's franchises in the Denver area. Shaquille O'Neal, Hall of Fame basketball center, has fifteen Auntie Anne's franchises under his belt. Whether these men are touting creamy lattes, gooey pizzas, or cinnamon sugar pretzels drenched in butter, you can bet the food is *perceived* as good, because of the athletes who stand behind them.

An additional marketing trick is taking a few items and projecting their goodness to the whole brand. This may not be intentional on Subway's part, but by touting the benefits of their *healthy choice line* that offers "6 grams of fat or less on a 6 inch sub," people who don't do their homework, assume that that *all* their subs are healthy. Many of Subway's menu selections *are* better than most of their rivals, *but* that's if you order lean meats on a whole grain roll and then load up on lots of veggies *without the zigzagging streams of mayo and dressings,* which is how the now famous Jared did it. [3] Jared lost his huge amount of weight by eating a 6-inch turkey sub for lunch and a 12-inch Veggie Delite® sub for dinner with *no cheese, no mayo* and *no salad dressing.* On the other hand, if you eat a foot-long line of fatty cold cuts, cheese, mayo, and salad dressing, the sub's grand total can be well over 1,000 calories, over 50 grams of fat, and over 2,000 mg of salt. Not so good, no matter how high you pile the lettuce.

Another phenomenon is when food is perceived as healthy or low-calorie, such as the "100 calorie" snacks. Many people not only eat more of them, but they often reward themselves with a high calorie drink or dessert, which negates the benefit of the low-cal food.

The easiest way to prevent deception is to do the homework and **read the label before it hits the table**. Here are a few more tips on interpreting labels and lingo.

- ✓ If the label says it's healthy, it doesn't mean the food is low in calories.
- ✓ If the word fruit is on the label, it doesn't mean there's fruit in the food or drink. It may be flavorings instead.
- ✓ If a package says "organic" or "low cholesterol" or "natural," it doesn't mean it's low in calories or healthy in *all* areas.
- ✓ If it takes a chemist to decode the ingredients or you can't pronounce most of the words, you probably shouldn't be eating it.
- ✓ If you eat more than the food's recommended serving size, remember to double, triple, or quadruple the number to get a more accurate total.
- ✓ If the label says the food is healthy in one area, it doesn't mean it's healthy in all areas. To compensate for the removal of fat, producers often add extra sugar or salt to make up the difference in taste.

- ✓ If a food lists sugar (sucrose) or its derivative (brown sugar, corn sweetener, corn syrup, dextrose, high-fructose corn syrup, or raw sugar), *as the first* or second ingredient on the label, it should be eliminated from the diet or eaten in moderation.

KNOW YOUR ABCs

As a person must know the basics of grammar and punctuation to write well, a person should also have a basic understanding of vitamins and minerals in order to eat well. When you see what these nutrients can do for you, it's more likely that you'll eat the foods that contain them. I've only included a few of the major players, since there are many more vitamins and minerals aside from the ones listed here.

As you read through this section, you will see how many of these disorders and illnesses can be prevented or minimized by eating healthy foods. Ironically, some of the most malnourished people in the United States are those who are overweight or obese, because they eat poor quality foods.

If nutrients build up the immune system and every cell of the body, then it stands to reason that a lack of nutrients can break down these same systems and cells. Therefore, even though being frail or hardy is due in part to genetics and activity levels, it is extremely dependent on whether or not a person eats nutritious or inferior food.

While reading the following lists, you may discover what ails you, or your child, or someone else you know. These are just a few examples of what can possibly happen if vitamins or minerals are lacking in the diet. I've also included a few examples of food sources in each category that assist in improving health. There are also many more food choices besides the ones listed here.

A lack of **Vitamin A** may be the cause of vision problems, susceptibility to infection, poor growth, and skin problems such as acne. Vitamin A (beta-carotene) is an antioxidant that zaps free radicals (those bad boys that damage cells and age the body). The best sources of Vitamin A are sweet potatoes, carrots, spinach, squash, dried apricots, cantaloupe, red peppers, and mangoes.

A lack of **Thiamin (B_1)** may be the cause of lack of energy, skin problems, nervous system disorders, apathy, confusion, short-term memory loss, irritability, and muscle weakness. The best sources of thiamin are sunflower seeds, fortified cereals, whole grain foods, lean pork, peas, and beans.

A lack of **Riboflavin (B_2)** may be the cause of inflammation of the mouth, tongue or throat, skin problems, eye and nervous system problems, confusion, and headaches. The best sources of riboflavin are fortified cereals, whole grain foods, cheese, almonds, yogurt, milk, eggs, spinach, and lean beef.

A lack of **Niacin (B_3)** may be the cause of lack of appetite, weakness, or a red, rough rash that worsens in the sunlight. The best sources of niacin are lean beef, tuna, poultry, fortified cereals, whole grain foods, peanuts, and salmon.

A lack of **Pantothenic Acid (B_5)** may be the cause of headache, fatigue, poor muscle coordination, and gastrointestinal disorders. The best sources of pantothenic acid are lean beef, chicken, milk, oats, potatoes, fortified cereals, whole grain foods, eggs, broccoli, sunflower seeds, yogurt, and peanuts.

A lack of **Vitamin B_6** may be the cause of confusion, convulsions, depression, red, dry, itchy, scaly skin and scalp or susceptibility to infection. A study on Vitamin B_6 has shown promise in improving behaviors in children with ADHD. [4] The best sources of Vitamin B_6 are fortified cereals and whole grain foods, lean beef, pork, fish, poultry, potatoes, spinach, bananas, sunflower seeds, garbanzo beans, avocados, and peanuts.

A lack of **Vitamin B_{12}** may be the cause of tingling or numbness in the legs, inability to concentrate, loss of memory, dementia, and disorientation. The best sources of Vitamin B_{12} are seafood, beef, poultry, fortified cereals, yogurt, milk, ham and eggs.

A lack of **Vitamin C** (ascorbic acid) may be the cause of fatigue, tiny red spots (hemorrhages) on the back of the arms and legs, bruising (easily), bleeding gums, nosebleeds, slow wound healing, and joint pain. Vitamin C is an antioxidant that zaps free radicals. It also aids in the absorption of iron. The best sources of Vitamin C are citrus fruits and fruit juices, Brussels sprouts, strawberries, red peppers, kiwi, broccoli, and tomatoes.

A lack of **Vitamin D** may be the cause of soft or weak bones, kidney disease, diabetes, lung disorders, and gastrointestinal problems. Studies have also found that a Vitamin D deficiency may result in an increased risk of autoimmune diseases, muscle weakness and pain, depression, thyroid conditions, psoriasis, and Alzheimer’s disease.

Vitamin D has shown promise in reducing inflammation in asthma, rheumatoid arthritis, multiple sclerosis, and Crohn's disease. It can also enhance mental clarity and memory function. The best sources of Vitamin D are (limited) exposure to sunshine, salmon, sardines, tuna, fortified milk, and egg yolks. Vitamin D deficiencies are *extremely* common, especially in people who live in places where sunshine is limited during the year.

A lack of **Vitamin E** may be the cause of a weakened immune system, muscle weakness, or vision problems. Vitamin E is an antioxidant that zaps free radicals. It may also shield the body against cardiovascular disease, arthritis, and cancer. Some of the best sources of Vitamin E are sunflower oil, safflower oil, canola oil, dry roasted sunflower seeds, dry roasted almonds, whole grains (wheat germ), and peanut butter.

A lack of **Vitamin K** may be the cause of excessive bleeding. Major sources of Vitamin K are dark leafy greens, asparagus, Brussels sprouts, broccoli, cabbage, and yogurt.

A lack of **Folate (Folic Acid)** may be the cause of anemia, diarrhea, weakened immune system, and birth defects. Folate is essential for tissue growth and cell function. The best sources of folate are dark leafy greens, fortified cereals and whole grain breads, asparagus, lentils, oranges, and broccoli.

MINING FOR MINERALS

The human body contains a treasure trove of the same elements that are abundant in the earth. All the minerals we need to stay healthy are found in the soil, or found in plants that get their minerals from the soil, or found in animals that eat the plants that are dependent on the soil. A few of them are listed here:

A lack of **Calcium** may be the cause of stunted growth in children, weak or soft bones and teeth, muscle spasms and cramps, and irregular heartbeat. The best sources of calcium are salmon, sardines, yogurt, fortified orange juice, milk, cheese, almonds, broccoli, and eggs.

A lack of **Magnesium** may be the cause of irregular heartbeat, weakness, muscle pain or spasms, twitches, disorientation, nausea, sleep disturbances, seizures, leg cramps, headaches, PMS, depression, lack of energy, irritability, decreased attention span, and mental confusion. A lack of magnesium may also contribute to ADHD. [5] Many metabolic functions are dependent on magnesium to do their jobs. The best sources of magnesium are almonds, cashews, peanut butter, sunflower seeds, dark leafy greens, garbanzo, kidney, and black beans, oatmeal, whole grain foods, potatoes, squash, brown rice, lentils, meats, milk, yogurt, eggs, and bananas.

A lack of **Iron** may be the cause of pale skin and lips, fatigue, shortness of breath, the inability to concentrate, infections, and behavioral disturbances in children. It may also be a contributing factor to symptoms of ADHD. [6] The best sources of iron are beef, venison, poultry, salmon, shrimp, ham, fortified cereals, molasses, spinach, and lentils.

Vitamin C foods should be eaten with iron-rich foods to aid in the absorption of iron. Caffeine blocks iron absorption. Therefore, avoid drinking coffee, tea, or cola drinks an hour before or after eating iron rich foods. According to the World Health Organization, iron deficiency anemia is the most widespread nutritional problem in the world, affecting over two *billion* people.

A lack of **Potassium** may be the cause of fatigue, muscle weakness or cramps, confusion, low blood-pressure, and irregular heartbeat. Potassium balances the harmful effects of too much sodium. The best sources of potassium are kidney and white beans, baked potatoes, yogurt, avocadoes, squash, oranges, cantaloupe, bananas, lima beans, dark leafy greens, sweet potatoes, and tomato products.

A lack of **Zinc** may be a cause of slow or poor growth and development, diarrhea, impaired immune function, slow healing, acne, hair loss, loss of taste and smell. A lack of zinc may also be the cause of ADHD. (Many children diagnosed with ADHD have low levels of zinc.) [7] The best sources of zinc are beef, pork, lamb, poultry, shellfish, whole grains, peanuts, beans, yogurt, cheese, sunflower seeds, and fortified cereals.

NOTE: Synthetic vitamins and minerals bought over-the-counter may contribute to overall health and help prevent deficiencies, but never take or give high doses of supplements to your children without a doctor's approval and supervision, since a few of them can be toxic in high doses.

HOME RUN! THE HEALING POWER OF FOOD

If the previous section wasn't enough to convince you that healthy food is medicine, here are a few more examples to prove the power and benefits of super foods.

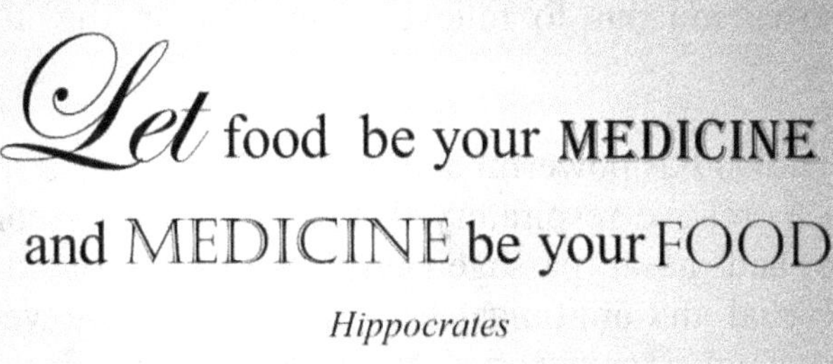

Garlic has been used for medical purposes for thousands of years, but it wasn't until Louis Pasteur placed garlic in a Petri dish of bacteria and noted that the bacteria died, that the antiseptic properties in garlic were proven. (Garlic contains acillin, such as in peni*cillin*.) Garlic also fights bacteria in the intestines, reduces cholesterol, lowers blood pressure, acts as an anticoagulant, and inhibits the growth of cancers and tumors.

Yogurt with probiotics (live acidophilus) are good bacteria that "eat" harmful bacteria in the intestines. When antibiotics destroy both good and bad bacteria during an illness, yogurt replenishes the good organisms to create a healthy balance again. Probiotics have also been used to prevent and to heal diarrhea, vaginal yeast infections, and urinary tract infections.

Fruits, vegetables, beans, and whole grains contain phytochemicals that interfere with the cancer producing process by blocking the development of tumors and ridding the body of harmful chemicals. Find out more at www.cancer.org.

Green tea has shown promise in blocking, inhibiting or diminishing cancer cells. It may also prevent and heal damage from sun exposure, by killing free radicals that harm cells.

Jalapeño peppers are natural chest expectorants that thin and loosen mucous to relieve congestion in the nose and lungs.

Horseradish has powerful antioxidant properties. It has been known to relieve respiratory distress by clearing congested sinuses and nasal passageways. It is also touted as an antibacterial and antifungal food that may also lower blood pressure and increase resistance to cancer. Even small amounts have been proven to be extremely beneficial to health.

Oranges, peppermint, and parsley contain the nutrient apigenin, which has shown promise in killing cancer cells.

Fish (salmon, sardines, and herring), walnuts, and flaxseed contain omega-3 fatty acids that work like aspirin to lower inflammation in the body. Omega-3s also strengthen and support the cardiovascular system, boost overall brain health and function, and may prevent or lessen the symptoms of Alzheimer's disease, dementia, asthma, Rheumatoid arthritis, lupus, and depression. A lack of omega-3 fatty acids may be a cause of eczema, psoriasis, sleep disturbances, ADHD, [8] and muscle pain.

Chicken noodle soup (homemade) helps soothe upper respiratory cold symptoms. The medicinal value is not just the steam that thins and moves mucus along, but also the antibiotic-like property of allicin in onions and garlic, and the anti-inflammatory property found in celery and carrots (Vitamin A).

THE REAL DEAL VERSUS FAUX FOOD

There is a defining line between nutritious and hazardous foods. Most of the time the distinction is clear, but other times the contrast is blurred. Deceptive marketers are the biggest proponents who smudge the line in an attempt to confuse consumers and keep them from knowing the truth.

Faux food
manufacturers and marketers
ARE MORE CONCERNED
about making money
than they are about your child's health.

Faux food contains a real food name or appears to be real, but provides little or no nutritional value. Faux food is an imitation of the real deal. It contains worthless calories that often lead to weight gain and health loss. Just as two objects cannot occupy the same space, the same holds true for what we eat. When your child fills up on faux food, it leaves little room for the real deal.

Ideally, ninety percent of what children eat should be high-quality, nutrient dense, whole food. The problem is the number is often reversed when the faux foods become the major items on the menu.

Having a real food name on the box or the bag, such as *fruit* snacks, *cheese* puffs, or *fish* sticks, doesn't mean that the product contains enough of that food to benefit health. Surprisingly, much of the food that producers sell under the guise of being healthy is really faux food. They perform this trick by twisting information and fooling buyers into believing their food is a quality product.

This trickery is done by illusion and distraction, as they advertise, "Look! No cholesterol," while hoping you don't see the hand behind their back that says, "Ooops! Contains loads of fat or sugar." Deceptive marketing hinders our ability to decipher misleading lingo. When this happens, innocent consumers buy their inferior products.

Once you understand the catchphrases marketers use, you can see how they disguise their unhealthy products with buzzwords that most people don't understand. Such is the case when they say fully hydrogenated oil, which is another word for saturated fat.

Another ploy is to break down an ingredient to make it appear as though there is less of it. If sugar is the main ingredient, manufacturers will often divvy it up into three or four smaller groups, and then use the different names of sugar (words ending in -ose), so sugar doesn't appear as the main ingredient, when in fact it really is, if all the various forms of sugar were combined. Deceptive marketing? Yup.

In all the following examples, the bad ingredients outweigh the "good" that the producers peddle. There are no redeeming qualities in these foods, therefore, they should be limited or eliminated from your child's diet, pronto!

THE OLD SWITCHEROO

Fish sticks contain real fish, but the amount is so minute that it's hard to find the little fella buried in the breading. Take one apart and see for yourself. Better choices are broiled, baked, or grilled fish fillets and steaks or water-packed canned tuna and salmon.

Pancake syrup contains no maple syrup. Nada! None! Not a lick! And that's because *pure maple* syrup is expensive. If it's pure maple syrup it must be labeled that it's the real deal. If it's not then it's an imitation. When the label says *Pancake Syrup* or *Original Syrup* (whatever that's supposed to mean), it's almost *entirely* corn syrup and high fructose corn syrup with a smidgen of maple flavoring. The average popular pancake syrups contain 42 grams of sugar (10½ teaspoons) in less than one-fourth cup.

Healthier toppings for whole grain pancakes, waffles, and French toast would be a light drizzle of *pure* maple syrup or a bit of 100% fruit spread or fresh fruit instead. Even a light dusting of powdered sugar would be a huge improvement over the golden flow.

Cheese Puffs are made of corn meal and oil and then coated with cheese seasonings, flavorings, and salt. Thirteen curls contain 150 calories, 10g of fat, and 300mg salt. Hardly worth the fluorescent orange fingers. Switch to Wheat Thins or corn tortillas in moderation for a crunchy snack. Serve carrot chips or carrots cut into "coins" for another crunchy substitute.

Fruit snacks and roll-ups contain no real fruit and very little fruit juice. They are made of sugar, fruit flavorings, and depending on the brand, carnauba wax and yellow dye 5. Carnauba wax makes fruit snacks shiny like a new car or polished floors and shoes. And that's because they use the same wax to get that glossy sheen. Carnauba wax, like paraffin, which is found in cheap chocolate and chewing gum, has been labeled safe for consumption. Regardless, would you chew on a candle or snack on car wax just because it was fruit flavored?

The yellow dye 5 found in fruit snacks may also cause allergic reactions, hyperactivity, and possibly cancer. Trade them in for dehydrated fruit for a similar chewy sweet treat. If you buy dried fruit choose organic and unsulfured products.

Non-dairy Whipped Topping lists water, tropical oils and high fructose corn syrup as the first three ingredients, all of which are whipped up together with a dollop of dairy and a slew of unpronounceable ingredients. No cream is involved in this product. If you do indulge in a whipped topping, use real whipped cream or whipped coconut cream in moderation instead.

Banana Chips are loaded with fat. This is because they are dried and then deep fried to give them their crunchy texture. The "fruit" that you assume is good is really bad for you. One particular brand in the produce aisle stated that a ½ cup serving of banana chips contained a whopping 10 grams of saturated fat! This is equivalent to the saturated fat in one Big Mac burger. Ten grams is over half your child's daily allowance! The easy solution is to dehydrate your own bananas or swap banana chips for real bananas. Add them to cereals and smoothies or slice them onto peanut butter sandwiches as a natural sweetener.

Strawberry Toaster Tarts contain little to no fruit or fiber, but they do contain almost four teaspoons of sugar in each pastry. A better choice would be a slice of whole grain toast with a bit of 100% fruit spread for more fiber and half the sugar.

Yogurt covered raisins and pretzels. Most people know that raisins, pretzels, and yogurt contain little or no fat, but are deceived by producers when these same foods are changed to make them more appealing. The food that is healthy in its natural state becomes unhealthy when fat and sugar are the main ingredients. Yogurt covered fruits, nuts, and pretzels are no better for you than chocolate covered fruits, nuts, and pretzels.

For example, according to Supertracker.usda.gov, one cup of yogurt covered mini-pretzels contains 11 grams of *saturated* fat and 391 calories. That's over half your child's daily saturated fat allowance. (Pretzels alone are 152 calories and contain almost no fat.) The numbers are similar for yogurt covered raisins.

The protein, calcium and live acidophilus found in real yogurt are also missing from these sugar and oil-based coatings. Step away from the yogurt covered raisins, and eat real raisins and real low-fat plain yogurt mixed with raw honey and fresh fruit instead.

The damage done by eating faux food is not just that it's unhealthy. It's that faux food is taking the place of high fiber foods and foods rich in vitamins and minerals. If your children are eating junky fluff, there is little room or desire for the good stuff.

Now repeat after me: "Faux food producers care more about making money than they do about my child's health." Remember this mantra when making food choices. Producers add fat, sugar, white flour, and salt to hook people on their products. If they really cared about your child's well-being, they would close their doors and fold up shop or change their products to make their foods more suitable for consumption.

THE OPPONENTS

Sugar, unhealthy fats, salt, and starchy white foods are the biggest opponents of ideal weight and excellent health. Controlling or overcoming these four foes, the Sugar Babes, the Fat Cats, the Salty Dogs, and the Gooey Guys, takes time, effort, practice and determination, just as it would to beat a rival in a rigorous sport.

So why take on this Goliath-like challenge? Because your family's health and quality of life are at stake. Studies have shown that when rats were given unlimited access to the opposing teams, especially the Sugar Babes, they had the same brain buzz as a person who snorted a line of cocaine. Over time they built up a tolerance, so in order to get the same "high" or pleasurable feeling, they had to eat even more of these same types of food (especially sugar-filled food). And like all addictions, it became more difficult to break the cycle the longer it continued. The chilling part is this rat habit and addiction, can becomes our habit and addiction, if we consume these same food. [9]

Addicted? Yes. Studies prove that this is true. If you don't believe it, try taking it away. Quit cold turkey and see what happens. Headaches, irritability, cravings and depression abound. It's better to wean your kids away to avoid the shock of withdrawal. Limit treats, eliminate soda, and gradually cut back on sugar.

OPPONENT 1: THE SUGAR BABES

In order to win the game, you have to know your opponents and how to keep score. If you don't know what you're up against, you won't know how to play. So grab some paper and a pen, and I'll show you how to tally the totals.

First, gather up a few obvious sources of sugar. Look in your refrigerator, freezer, and cupboards for soda, jams, syrups, cookies, donuts, candy, or ice cream, and then write down the name of the food and the number of sugar grams listed on the label. Do this with each item. If you usually eat two or three times the recommended serving size, double or triple the number to get an accurate sum. (The serving size is usually at the top of the label.)

Next, with pen and pad still in hand, check a few foods that you regularly eat but *would not expect to contain much sugar.* These items look like ketchup, barbeque sauce, flavored coffees, and honey-roasted peanuts. After you collect the items and data, do the math again, remembering to double or triple the amount of sugar grams, if you normally eat more.

Now pick out the foods that you usually eat in one day and then add these numbers together. When you are finished, take the total number of grams of sugar, and then divide it by four. The quotient is how many teaspoons of sugar you have eaten in one day.

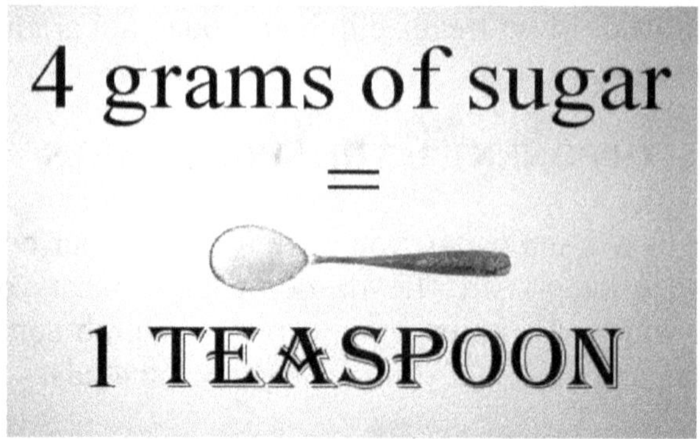

(g ÷ 4 = teaspoons of sugar)

Always divide the total number of sugar grams by 4 to see how many teaspoons of sugar are in a product.

Okay, so what about it? What do these numbers mean? Government based nutrition sites recommend that women limit their sugar consumption to 6 teaspoons a day. Yep, you read that right. Six measly teaspoons of sugar a day. A man is allowed a little bit more at 9 teaspoons a day. Children should limit their sugar intake to 5 teaspoon a day for girls, and 6 teaspoons a day for boys. (Be sure to write these numbers down on your notecards.)

This isn't very much allowable sugar, but if you want to feel amazing and have more energy, while losing weight and gaining health in the process, then sugar has to go, or at least be doled out in small measures.

Visions of sugarplums dancing through your child's head isn't just a sweet Christmas dream, it could become a lifetime nightmare. We've also heard Mary Poppins sing, "A spoonful of sugar makes the medicine go down," so it can't be all bad, right? It all sounds good, but it really isn't healthy for you or your children. Too much sugar on a daily basis erodes the body and leads to obesity and disease. Refined white sugar has no redeeming qualities whatsoever as you are about to discover.

FOOD WITH ATTITUDE

In the mid-1960s, my mom exercised along with the "godfather of fitness," Jack LaLanne, on television. Even then as a young girl, I was amazed at the man's vim, vigor and fit physique.

Jack was a pioneer in the fitness and nutrition field. Yet, when he was just a young boy, he was a self-proclaimed "sugarholic," a "junk food junkie," and troublemaker at school because of his poor diet. Jack said that sweets and junk food made him sick, weak, and mean. His nutritional deficiencies also riddled his skin with acne and boils.

The turning point in Jack's life came when he was fifteen years old. After hearing a nutritionist speak about the harmful effects of sugar and junk food, he began eating healthy and exercising faithfully. A short time later, this "problem child" evolved into a top high school athlete. Jack Lalane continued living this astounding lifestyle by doing incredible feats of strength and endurance well into his old age. He died at the age of 96. [10]

Black Teeth

Before modern dentistry came on the scene the effects of sugar were obvious. Hundreds of years ago, most people could neither attain, nor afford sugar even when it was available. There weren't many photos of smiling faces to behold, or research concerning the effects of sugar on teeth. Unless, of course, you were the queen, who could both acquire and afford the white wonder.

During the reign of Queen Elizabeth I, sugary foods flowed freely. The queen didn't know that sugar was potent enough to erode her teeth, so her love of sweets eventually lead to the demise of her pearly whites, when cavities turned her teeth black and missing in action. [11]

Too much sugar still rots teeth, but today when cavities do occur, we have dentists who drill and fill them, or fluoride in water, toothpaste, and mouthwash to prevent tooth decay. But the same damage that ravaged teeth still damages the bones and body, even though we may not see the effects right away.

Fatty Liver

Refined sugar and high fructose corn syrup are both simple sugars that are filtered through the liver and then eventually dispensed as fuel when needed. If too much sugar accumulates in the liver and the glycogen store is full, all excess incoming calories *from any source of food* are then *converted to fat* and then stored as fat.

Since fat doesn't discriminate where it resides, it's distributed and stored *everywhere*, *including* the liver and other organs. Internal organs padded with fat make them less efficient, but when the liver is surrounded by fat on the outside and speckled with fat on the inside, the filtration system gums up like clogged holes in a strainer. Over time, if there is no dietary improvement, this fatty liver may turn into *non-alcoholic fatty liver disease* (NAFLD).

In severe cases, a fatty liver can also become scarred. A fatty scarred liver is just another way to say cirrhosis of the liver. Shocking? Absolutely! Especially since the liver is the largest internal organ and filtration system in the body that we obviously need to survive. Plug the filter up with fat and scar tissue and the system can't cleanse and regulate the body properly. [12]

Type 2 Diabetes

The liver also plays a part in Type 2 diabetes. Many people believe that sugar is the cause of this dreaded enemy, but it's not the lone foe. It is the fat gained from eating too much sugar and bad fat, or too many calories in general, that can lead to diabetes. A fatty liver cannot "read" insulin signals, and therefore it cannot regulate blood-sugar properly. Not only that, but this sugar and fat dynamic duo is also the leading cause of almost all obesity related diseases such as heart disease, high blood pressure, cancer, and stroke.

You may not be concerned about these diseases when a child is young (although many children are affected by them), but tastes and preferences created at an early age become ingrained tastes and preferences as adults. Thirty years ago, Type 2 diabetes was rarely seen in children. Today, one-in-every three children have been diagnosed with it.

The plan for managing Type 2 diabetes is the same plan for prevention: Increase physical activity and decrease sugar and bad fat from the diet. If this information isn't enough to convince you that sugar should be limited or eliminated in your child's life, check out the Pop Flies and Line Drives that follow.

POP FLIES AND LINE DRIVES

Everything your children eat or drink influences their appetite, behavior, and emotions. Consuming foods that cause Pop Flies and Line Drives will affect how hungry or full they feel, how tired or energetic they feel, how irritable or content they feel, or how foggy or clear they think.

A pop fly is a ball hit high while not traveling far laterally. What goes up must come down like Pop Flies or sugar spikes. Knowing the truth about blood-sugar levels can save you a lot of headaches, confusion, illnesses, compulsive over-eating, and even your life.

Sugar spikes and dips, and stable blood sugar, refer to how quickly or how slow sugar reaches the intestines to be absorbed into the blood. The vertical spikes and dips in the following charts represent blood sugar levels after eating *simple carbohydrates* such as refined sugar or corn sweeteners (sodas, sugary drinks, candy, syrups, jellies, jams, etc.), and refined *white* grains (flour, rice, pasta, cakes, cookies, crackers, muffins, donuts, etc.).

If a high fiber food, protein, or good fat are not eaten at the same time, to counterbalance the effects of these refined foods, the Pop Flies become even more pronounced, and blood sugar skyrockets then plummets, to produce the feelings mentioned on the chart.

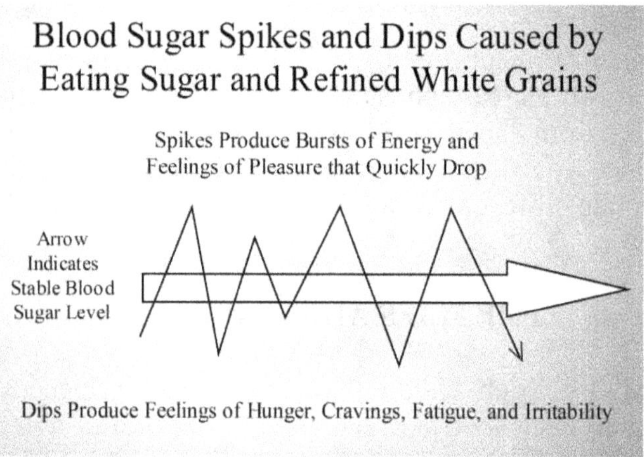

The immediate effects of too much sugar or refined white grains are that most children become hyper or "wired" and then crash. Spikes in blood sugar send out a surge of pleasure and energy, which sound great if you're gloomy or tired, but the quick mood enhancer and energy rush doesn't last very long. Soon thereafter the opposite affect kicks in, when the blood sugar level dips below the stable line of satisfaction.

Dips often create feelings of fatigue, brain fog, irritation, frustration, confusion, anxiety, whining, or weepiness. Further dips in blood sugar may also lead to feelings of sadness, depression, agitation, aggression, outbursts of anger, a combative attitude, compulsive overeating, or feelings of famish to the point where the hands may shake. (Shakiness may also be due to a caffeine surge and crash.)

Simple carbohydrate foods and drinks have the potential to leave your child feeling giddy to grumpy and then hungry again, all in a very short time. These simple carbohydrates also create cravings for more of these same mood foods to spike blood sugar levels up to their previous highs, in order to feel "good" again. Thus the vicious cycle continues as the excess calories stick around to be stored as fat in the liver and the body.

There's also an unusual paradox amid this whole rollercoaster of emotions: Most emotional eaters believe that they eat when they are emotional (and it's true). Yet it may be more accurate to say that *what they are eating is creating the emotions that they are feeling*, which causes them to eat the wrong foods again, to raise the blood sugar level up once more to recreate the good feeling again. You may want to reread the previous two paragraphs to fully understand this concept: Emotional eaters often *feel* the way they do because of what they have or haven't eaten.

The following chart shows how lean protein, healthy fats, whole grain foods, and high fiber veggies and fruit play out. As you can see, rather than a sudden pop fly, there is a calmer, consistent line drive.

Blood Sugar Waves After Eating
High Fiber Foods, Protein, and Good Fats

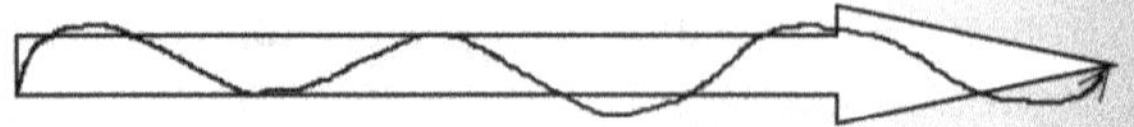

Arrow Indicates Blood Sugar Range that Creates a Feeling of Fullness, Satisfaction, and Well-being

The white arrow represents the range where blood sugar stability occurs. The wavy line within the white arrow fluctuates slightly, but the horizontal hit stays within the stable range after eating the following types of foods:

1. Low-fat dairy products and eggs.

2. High fiber foods: beans, peas, lentils, whole grains, vegetables, and fruit.

3. Lean meats and lean cuts of meat: fish, skinless chicken and turkey, beef, venison, pork.

4. Healthy fats in moderation: nuts and seeds, avocados, canola oil, olives and olive oil, coconut oil, sesame oil, and flaxseed oil.

These hearty foods keep kids feeling full longer and help keep their blood sugar and emotions in check. Lean protein, high fiber foods and good fats slow down digestion and absorption to control or prevent Pop Flies. You probably know that fruits, veggies, and dairy products contain small amounts of sugar, but these are *natural* sugars that metabolize well and assimilate slower. This is also because they contain fiber, fat, or protein, all of which prevent the sugar from making a beeline to the small intestines and then the blood.

Understanding how blood sugar works and then making healthy food choices will help your children think more clearly, it will help them rein in their emotions, and it will help them feel less hungry all the time. High fiber foods, lean protein, and good fat are the tickets to health, wellness, and weight loss.

THE BASES ARE LOADED

Monitoring a daily sugar quota is nearly impossible. The truth is that it's difficult to stay completely away from sugar, because it's found in a ton of stuff that we eat and drink every day. Therefore, it's best to tackle the biggest offenders, to limit or eliminate the amount of sugar our kids are spooning down their throats. The biggest sources of sugar-filled foods that children frequently consume are soft drinks, candy, cakes, cookies, pies, and sweetened cereals.

Advertisers are after your children and they woo them accordingly. They entice them with commercials that promise fun, friends, and magical experiences, if they eat their products. This media brainwashing goes on right under innocent little noses while tiny tots are engrossed in their favorite television shows. And in our parental love and desire to make our children happy, we often give in and buy these sweet, yet unhealthy treats.

Just as two objects cannot occupy the same space, a child will not receive the healthy benefits of fiber, vitamins and minerals that are found in whole, real food, if his or her appetite is spoiled by sugary sodas, candy, and rainbow-colored cereals.

I stated earlier that faux food manufacturers care more about making money than they do your child's health, but this is also true for food vendors at circuses, carnivals, fairs, and fast-food restaurants.

Again, if these people really cared about your children's health, weight, teeth, and emotional well-being, they would fold-up shop, or do a complete overhaul, to make their products healthier. But most of them don't. And that's because sugar is an addictive moneymaker, just like a drug. Once hooked, people buy it.

So here's the scoop on where to find those addictive white crystals.

STRIKE ONE! SODA, PUNCH, AND OTHER DRINKS

Sugary drinks are one of the biggest contributors to obesity and disease. The main ingredients in soda, fruit drinks, and punch are water and sugar with a touch of flavoring and fizz. Some producers add a 100% dose of Vitamin C to make their products *appear* healthier. Aside from that they provide no nutritional value.

If the word drink, punch, or cocktail is on the label, you can bet that it's full of sugar. If the label doesn't say 100% *fruit juice*, it's usually about 90% sugar water, additives and 10% or less of real fruit juice.

Many soft drink producers are wising up and reducing their sugar content in order to appear healthier. A few are lightening their sugar load by adding artificial sweeteners to their drinks. Sounds a bit deceptive unless you know what you're looking for on the ingredient label (more on this shortly). Many more will soon jump on the bandwagon as consumers become more informed and stop buying their syrupy drinks.

Ghastly Stats

The following are a few eye-openers. If you check these numbers for yourself and see that the sugar in the products are less than stated here, the producers may have reduced the sugar content because of consumer awareness and outrage, or they may have added artificial sweeteners to their products since the publication of this book.

12 teaspoons = ¼ cup of sugar
24 teaspoons = ½ cup of sugar
36 teaspoons = ¾ cup of sugar
48 teaspoons = 1 cup of sugar

Brace yourself before you read these mind-boggling numbers: One 12 to 20 ounce serving of soda, Snapple, sweetened tea, lemonade, Gatorade, Arizona, Sunny D, or Hawaiian Punch may contain anywhere between 10 to 20 *or more* teaspoons of sugar, depending on the product and its serving size.

A parent would never think of pouring a dozen teaspoons of sugar into a glass of water, stirring it up, and then handing it to a child to drink, but many unintentionally do when they allow them to consume these products. Here are a few more double-digit examples.

- Pepsi (12 ounce) 10¼ teaspoons of sugar.
- Jolt (23.5 ounces) 23½ teaspoons of sugar.
- Mountain Dew (20 ounces) 19¼ teaspoons of sugar.
- SOBE green tea (20 ounces) 12¾ teaspoons of sugar.

- Sunkist Pineapple Soda (20 ounces) 20¾ teaspoons of sugar.
- Rock Star Energy drink (16 ounces) 15½ teaspoons of sugar.
- Minute Maid Lemonade (20 ounces) 16¾ teaspoons of sugar.
- Cold Stone Cake and Batter Shake (large) 33¼ teaspoons of sugar.
- McDonald's chocolate shake (large) 30 teaspoons of sugar.
- Starbucks Peppermint White Chocolate Mocha with Whipped Cream (20 ounces) 18¾ teaspoons of sugar.

Notice that many of these drinks break down to *one teaspoon of sugar per ounce!* Some of these drinks contain less sugar, but others have even more!

Milkshakes not only contain a boatload of sugar, but also an avalanche of fat. Any beverage made with lemons usually contains a ton of sugar to counteract the sour taste. Any drink made with an ice cream base is guaranteed to contain a mountain of sugar and fat. Many foods that are high in sugar are also high in fat.

If you do nothing else but eliminate soda and other sugary drinks from your child's diet, you will be taking huge strides toward lowering their weight and improving their health. Children should not drink their calories unless they come from low-fat milk, healthy smoothies, or 100% fruit juices.

Kick Energy Drinks to the Curb

As long as we're in the drink department, here are a few facts about the caffeine in energy drinks. Caffeine is a drug. It's a legal addictive stimulant. And like any other drug, a person can build up a tolerance to it, so that over time more is needed to get the same effect as the previous jolt.

Caffeine works by stimulating nerve cells to release adrenaline which kicks up the heartbeat and speeds up breathing. Some energy drinks contain guarana (40 mg of caffeine per gram), a Brazilian cocoa seed, which is often left out of the caffeine tally on the ingredient label. Many energy drinks also contain mega doses of Vitamin B6 (over 8,000% of the daily value) and B12 (over 2,000% of the daily value). [13]

Many children are innocently consuming energy drinks and colas that contain enough caffeine to wreak havoc on their health. Many adolescents are deliberately consuming energy drinks and colas for a boost of energy or to stay awake to study for tests.

Research has found that adolescents who drink excessive amounts of colas and energy drinks experience an increase in blood pressure, heart palpitations, chest pains, hyperactivity, irritability, anxiety attacks, jitters, tremors, restlessness or insomnia.

Extremely high levels of caffeine in a child's system may require a trip to the emergency room. Heavy caffeine consumption in short periods of time has been linked to seizures, stroke, heightened states of frenzy, and even sudden death. [14]

Children who have medical conditions such as seizures, diabetes, heart irregularities, anxiety problems or those who are on medications should especially be wary of caffeine in their diets. Authorities agree that a safe daily dose of caffeine for an adolescent is **100 milligrams or less.**

So here is what you need to know: Brewed coffees, lattes, or mocha frappes (8 ounces) prepared at home or restaurants contain between 70 and 165 mg of caffeine.

Cola sodas (12 ounce can) contain anywhere between 18 and 55 mg of caffeine. Root beer contains the least amount, and Mountain Dew contains the most. Pepsi and Coke fall in the mid-30 mg range. A few more include:

- Hype (16 ounces) energy drink contains 160 mg of caffeine.

- 5-Hour energy drink (***2 ounces***) contains 207 mg of caffeine.

- Sunkist Orange Soda (20 ounces) contains 68 mg of caffeine.

- Rockstar Punched Guava (22 ounces) contains 330 mg of caffeine.

- Red Bull or Rock Star energy drinks (8 ounces) contains 80 mg of caffeine.

Although it's not a drink, Extra Strength Excedrin contains 130 mg of caffeine in two tablets. NoDoz maximum strength contains 200 mg in one tablet. Caffeine is also found in smaller doses in chocolate and tea. I mention this because of the possible combinations that, though unwittingly consumed, may still generate the negative effects of too much caffeine racing through the body.

High doses of caffeine also have a rebound effect. Once the caffeine kick wears off, many people feel lethargic, headachy, or foggy-headed. This may start the cycle over again in an attempt to relieve the withdrawal symptoms.

NOTE: As mentioned earlier, caffeine blocks the absorption of iron, which can lead to anemia.

STRIKE TWO! CANDY, CAKES, COOKIES, AND PIES

Candy is one of the biggest sources of concentrated sugar on the planet. Hard candy, cotton candy, candy canes, taffy, jelly beans, chocolates, sourballs, gumdrops, licorice, chewing gum, you name it. No matter what form it presents itself, the primary ingredient in candy is pure sugar. The following are just a few examples of how much sugar lurks in common treats.

- Jell-O (1 cup) 38g (9½ teaspoons sugar)
- Freeze pop (1 tube) 12g sugar (3 teaspoons)
- Skittles (2.17 ounce bag) 46g (11½ teaspoons sugar)
- Candy Corn (19 kernels) 28g (7 teaspoons sugar)
- Snickers (1 bar) 27g (6¾ teaspoons sugar)
- Dum Dums lollipops (3 tiny suckers) 11g (2¾ teaspoons sugar)
- Fruit *flavored* snacks or rollups (1 pouch) 12g (3 teaspoons sugar)
- Breyers Rocky Road ice cream (1 cup / 1 scoop) 30g (7½ teaspoons sugar)

Cakes, cookies, pies, pastries, cinnamon rolls, and donuts are the most common confections that children eat. This is where the Sugar Babes and the Gooey Guys merge and gain strength to overpower your child. More on this in the "Playoff" section.

Time Out! From Holidaze to Crazy Daze!

Every year we chew our way through Halloween candy, Thanksgiving pies, Christmas cookies, chocolate hearts and Easter Bunnies, and then birthday, graduation and wedding cakes. Then, there's after dinner desserts and ice cream socials, in-between each holiday fête. We're surrounded by treats at every turn. We can't seem to get away from them. It's like living in a gingerbread house where the walls are frosted with icing and adorned with lollipops and gumdrops, to be plucked and eaten whenever the desire so strikes.

Autumn sparks the season of overeating. Many people take a break from healthy living, especially during these three key months. Surely, it's because they feel it's hopeless to control. Many try to recoup their good intentions after the New Year by making resolutions, but most people feel they're fighting a losing battle and then give up after a few weeks. This mindset affects more adults than children, yet children are taking their cues from adults, and may someday follow suit.

So when will it end? It doesn't unless you do something different. Nothing changes if nothing changes, consistently, over time. If children partake in these festivities, as most of them usually do, they're consuming a *tremendous* amount of sugar and empty calories during their formative years.

Sugar begins by making you FEEL GOOD, but then it makes you **feel bad**, either because of the sugar dip blues and irritability, weight gain, or *disease*.

So how do we deal with the avalanche of candy? Hide it? Dole it out in little bits after they have eaten well? Throw it away? Maybe. If we ration it out in *very small measures,* it may not be as bad. I've done that at Christmastime and other holidays, but I've also done the following too: Instead of buying pounds of Easter candy for my daughters, I offered to buy new clothes or other gifts instead. And you know what? It worked. Voilà!

Your children may actually prefer a few little trinkets or toys, or a new pair of jeans, or movie passes, rather than chocolate rabbits and jelly beans. Give them a few pieces of candy for tradition sake if you must, but swap the rest for gifts instead.

Rather than trick-or-treating on Halloween offer alternatives: Better yet, take a trip to the skating rink, a trampoline park, or a place that offers laser tag. Coax them away from candy with books, small toys, plastic jewelry, stickers, sunglasses, or fake teeth. If they come home with hordes of chocolate, freeze as much of it as you can, and then ration it out in small doses *after they have eaten well.* Set a limit of two small pieces a day, such as one after lunch and one after supper. Another alternative is to save the candy that they favor, and throw the rest away.

If you do allow them to eat candy, don't let them eat it on an empty stomach. If they're hungry, they may eat four or more times the amount that they would normally eat. Their blood sugar will also skyrocket and fall like a signal flare.

You can also explain to them the harmful effects of sugar by saying something like, "I love you too much to feed that junk to you. It doesn't help you grow or keep you healthy and strong." I did this when I took my four year-old grandson to the circus. A vendor walked by hawking clouds of cotton candy, and my grandson innocently raised his hand to call him over. I felt terrible saying no, but I explained the reasons why, and I immediately offered to buy him something else instead, to which he happily agreed. At four-years old, he understood and took the better deal.

Yeah, yeah, I know. The circus only comes to town once a year, but the point is, there will always be some "special" occasion in any given month of the year, and if I can substitute a better choice for the worst choice, I'll do it. I also remind myself that love and fun are measured in other ways. Not by giving a child over one-fourth-cup of sugar, whipped up and stuffed in a plastic bag.

I would also feel worse seeing my candy-fed kids giddy and giggly one day, but then sick with a headache or stomachache or some other ailment another day, because their immune systems weren't strong enough to fight the latest flu. (The American Journal of Clinical Nutrition discovered that eating 25 teaspoons of sugar slowed down the ability of white blood cells to kill bacteria for up to 5 hours after eating the sweet stuff.) It's also sad to see overweight children being bullied or being stuck with needles or taking pills every day to control their depleted insulin because they're diabetic.

Healthy food increases a child's resistance to infections and ailments. Sugar depletes the immune system which leads to illness and disease. This is primarily because sugary foods take the place of nutritious foods, that support the body and makes it strong. If a person with a healthy immune system does become ill, he or she often experiences less intense symptoms and recovers more quickly than those who are weaker because of sweet treats and lack of nutrients.

Excessive amounts of sugar and fat do not equal love. Time and attention equals love.

Out of Bounds?

While limiting or eliminating sugar from your child's diet, you may wonder about artificial sweeteners. Are they safe? Yes? No? There are pros and cons from many sources, but the U.S. Food and Drug Administration has given their stamp of approval to the following artificial sweeteners after researching and finding them safe to consume as sugar substitutes. You will find these sweeteners under names such as sucralose (Splenda), saccharin (Sweet 'N Low, Sweet Twin, NectaSweet), neotame, and aspartame (NutraSweet and Equal).

Companies that make Little HUGS, Sunny D, Kool-aid Jammers, chocolate milk and other drinks that appeal to kids are wising up, because people are reading labels to make better choices about sugar. To keep sales high, many of these producers are now adding *sugar substitutes* to their products so they can market them as low-sugar. Look in your cupboard or refrigerator right now. You may unwittingly have some hiding in your home at this very moment, concealed under the guise of *sucralose* (Splenda), which coincidentally, looks a lot like *sucrose* (table sugar) if you don't read the label carefully.

Studies have concluded that the aforementioned substitutes are safe to consume, and that there are far more disease related deaths, as previously mentioned, due to eating refined white sugar and corn sweeteners. Experts agree that the *possible risks* from eating artificial sweeteners are far less, than the *probable danger* associated with eating refined sugar.

Limiting or eliminating sugar or switching to a sugar substitute lessens occurrences of spikes and dips and the diseases, such as Type 2 diabetes, heart disease, stroke, cancer, and hypertension, that are prone to those who are overweight,. Not to mention the stigma and discomfort of being overweight, which also interferes with quality of life for a child.

Since these substitutes are approved by the FDA and the National Cancer Institute, they are considered safe to use. It's your call.

NOTE: People with the hereditary disease phenylketonuria (PKU) should not consume aspartame.

STRIKE THREE! CEREAL AND GRANOLA BARS

Sugarcoated cereals that come in fun colors and that look and taste like cookies or candy often contain more sugar than cookies and candy. Most cereal manufacturers label a serving size as ¾ cup, which makes their sugar content seem lower than it actually is, because most older kids eat a heaping cup, or two, or three, which is more than the recommended serving size. Therefore, to see what your tykes are really taking in, double or triple the sugar grams listed on the label and then divide by four to see how many teaspoons of sweet stuff is floating in their bowls. Most of these types of cereal also contain very little fiber.

Although cereals that snap, crackle and pop upon adding milk or that boast the special letter K contain only one teaspoon of sugar per serving, there's nary a gram of fiber in the box. Cracklin' Oat Bran sounds like a healthy cereal, and although it contains 6 grams of fiber, which is good, it also contains 7 grams of fat, 3 grams of saturated fat, and 3½ teaspoons of sugar in a one cup serving.

Many granola bars are barely a notch above candy bars. Some are studded with chocolate chips and drizzled with caramel swirls, which brings their sugar and fat contents up to that of a candy bar status. Beware of organic or "natural" granola cereals too. Many of them are also high in sugar and fat.

A healthy alternative would be to make your own granola by mixing oats, nuts, seeds, and raisins together, and then storing the mix in an airtight container. Cook it like traditional hot oatmeal, or add milk, yogurt, and fruit to the granola and then refrigerate it overnight for cold oatmeal (muesli) in the morning.

Make your own trail mix instead of buying granola bars. Toss a handful of walnuts, almonds, peanuts, pumpkin or sunflower seeds, and raisins or dried berries together in an airtight container. Scoop a small amount into a Ziploc bag to carry as a kid-friendly snack on the go. If you do choose prepackaged granola bars or cereal, opt for the Kashi brand, but here again, read the labels. Healthy brands are not necessarily healthy across the board.

The best cereal choices are those that contain the least amount of sugar and fat and the most amount of fiber (at least 3g per serving) and vitamins. A *whole* grain should be the first ingredient listed on the label. Look for these five things when choosing cereal:

1. Low sugar
2. Low fat
3. Whole grains listed first
4. High fiber (3g or more per serving)
5. High in vitamins and minerals

A few examples of more nutritious cereals are regular Cheerios, Total, Chex, Shredded Wheat, Fiber One, Raisin Bran, and Kashi brands. Most of these whole grain cereals are enriched, so they also provide many vitamins and minerals that are often difficult to obtain in the average diet. Add sliced bananas or berries to sweeten things up, and you've added even more fiber and nutrients to your breakfast or snack.

NOTE: Nutritional numbers may change by the time you read this, as producers buckle under consumer outcry.

Bunt: A Little Hit

Sugar is sugar no matter what form it takes, but raw and dark honeys, maple syrup, and molasses are slightly beneficial because they contain small amounts of nutrients. Raw and dark honeys (buckwheat and sunflower) contain antioxidants that boost the immune system and zap free radicals. Honey contains a trace amount of hydrogen peroxide, which is why it was a perfect salve and sealer for wounds and skin diseases before modern medicine. [15]

This liquid gold also contains Vitamin B_6, Vitamin C, and riboflavin. Maple syrup contains small amounts of manganese, zinc, calcium, iron, and potassium. Molasses also contains small amounts of calcium, magnesium and iron.

Honey has been used as a sweetener and for medicinal purposes, for thousands of years. It's been found intact and still edible in Egyptian pyramids. The Bible mentions

Sampson eating wild honey and being refreshed. The Hebrew children were promised a land flowing with milk and honey. King David and John the Baptist both ate wild honey for pleasure and health benefits. The Word of God is even compared to honey.

Even though honey, maple syrup, and molasses contain more nutrients than refined sugar, they are still forms of sugar that can cause Pop Flies and dips, and they are still *concentrated forms of calories* that can cause weight gain, so they should be eaten in moderation.

YOU'RE THE COACH SO YOU'RE IN CHARGE!

As a parent you're in charge of what is purchased at the store, what is prepared at home, and how often food is ordered in or eaten out. If a child cries or has a tantrum in the store because you don't buy the usual candy, ice cream, or soda, so be it. Just smile, nod, and shrug at the wide-eyed customers. A few may nod and smile in return with mutual understanding.

Others may not be so sympathetic. Don't be intimidated by well-meaning people and buckle under at their sighs or their pitiful stares at your children, because they think you're being mean to them. Be strong and stand firm. You're not doing your brood any favors by feeding them a cart full of empty calories that can make them sick and diseased, or fat and bullied down the road.

When you reduce the sugar in your children's diet and when you incorporate the suggestions in this book, changes take place in their demeanor. Once the initial shock of withdrawal wears off, and blood sugar levels begin to stabilize, happier, more cooperative children often emerge. Not only that, but once they begin to lose weight (if needed), they may even thank you someday. Health is the obvious priority, but a child's self-image is also at stake.

Body image plays a major role in your child's level of confidence. Confidence plays a major role in your child's level of sociability. Sociability plays a major role in your child's level of popularity. It's a sad fact, but people judge other people by their appearance. Weight-based discrimination exists at all ages, but it especially affects a child's social life and a young adult's dating and future job opportunities.

Overweight children are also more prone to being teased or bullied by their peers. Help them overcome their weaknesses by practicing tough love. If at any time you feel yourself wavering and wanting to give into their tantrums, because you feel like you're being mean, by withholding sugary treats, remember Annie Sullivan. If you've read the book or seen the movie, *The Miracle Worker*, about the life of Helen Keller, you know what I am talking about.

The Keller family felt so sorry for their blind, deaf, mute daughter that they neither challenged her to grow, nor required respect or obedience from her, and therefore, she became a little tyrant. When Annie Sullivan came to work with Helen, the parents thought Annie was cruel because she required Helen to act with respect and behave in a civil manner.

In the midst of Helen's tantrums, she had also been inadvertently trained to misbehave. Whenever Helen acted up, someone stuffed a piece of cake into her mouth to calm her wild outbursts. This may have contributed to her unruly behavior, since the girl dearly loved sweets, and since sweets cause blood-sugar spikes-and-dips, along with their extreme emotions.

It was the unwavering stance and persistence on Annie's part (even amid lengthy, horrific tantrums) that led to the success of the child. Annie took matters into her own hands by eliminating appeasement (cake and coddling for negative behavior) and rerouting Helen's life down a more agreeable and productive path, where she not only to learned to communicate, but also behave in a respectable way.

From an outside perspective, it didn't look like Annie cared for Helen because of her firm stance. But Annie did care. She cared enough to use tough love in the child's life for her own good, and it worked. [16] Annie wrote a letter to a friend that said, "I am certain that obedience is the gateway through which knowledge, yes, and love, too, enter the mind of the child." Annie and Helen became best friends and companions until the time of Annie's death, 50 years later.

The bottom line is that if you want to build your child's health and raise their self-esteem, don't feel sorry for them or give in to their junk food demands. Don't feel that you're depriving them of something good, when in fact it's something bad for them. If you quit buying faux food, it won't make them love you less. In the long-run, it may make them love you more, if you replace the faux food with healthy food, your time and attention, small non-food gifts, and meaningful activities instead.

Remember Annie Sullivan.

HOW TO CREAM THE SUGAR BABES

Maybe you think this doesn't apply to your child, so a little sugar won't hurt. Well maybe, but let's do the math. If a teenager drinks one regular-sized can of soda every day, which contains 10 teaspoons of sugar, that's seventy teaspoons of sugar per week (about 6 cups of sugar per month), which adds up to 3,640 teaspoons (approximately 38 pounds) of sugar a year. To put this in perspective, next time you go to the grocery store, count off 9 ½ (4 pound) bags of sugar to get an idea of how much sugar is being filtered through your child's liver and absorbed into his bloodstream and then turned to fat in one year. Then, imagine how many more sacks there would be, if you added all the other sources of sugar to the pile.

Maybe you don't believe in giving a child soda, and that's great, but how about a couple cookies instead? After all, it's only two cookies a day. That doesn't sound like a lot, and it's not, but when combined with other sugary treats, they all add up. Yet these two daily cookies become 730 cookies, or 61 dozen cookies a year. To get an eye-estimate, imagine 730 half-inch thick cookies stacked atop each other on a gymnasium floor. These circular sweeties would reach the height of three basketball rims! Many children slam dunk even more cookies than these in a year, and when combined with cake, candy, gum, chocolate, soda, and ice cream, we're talkin' a lotta sugar, baby. I mean a lotta Sugar Babes.

Steal Second Base!

So how do you kick it, taper off, or control it? Wean yourself away or offer something else instead! You can't steal second base with your foot on first! You can't reach a higher goal until you leave your comfort zone. You can't get a dog to drop his bone until you offer a steak in its place. On the same token, you can't take a child's sweets away until you offer something else instead.

A cookie or candy may be an immediate reward and used on occasion to wean a child away from sugar, but it's your time and attention that bring pleasure to a child. Most children would prefer your focused attention while doing something fun or exciting or interesting rather than loading up on fatty food, soda, and candy. Finding activities that pique their interest and then doing them will help deter them from candy land. A slew of suggestions are found in the "I'm Bored!" section.

Beat the Sugar Babes at the Fruit Bowl!

The original fruit snacks. Nature's candy. Whatever clever name you call it, fruit contains natural sugars that help curb a child's cravings. Even though fruit contains natural sugar, the fiber slows down digestion to helps prevent spikes and dips. Fruit is also packed with antioxidants, vitamins and minerals.

Keep a large bowl of fresh fruit on the counter where your children can easily see it and eat it. Frozen fruit is also great to blend in smoothies or mix in yogurt. Use sliced bananas on peanut butter sandwiches or as a sweetener in cereals. Layer yogurt and berries in fancy glasses then top with chopped walnuts for a creamy sweet parfait-like treat.

100% fruit juice will also curb their desire for sweets, but serve it in moderation. Experts agree that one 8 ounce glass a day is plenty. Although it contains natural sugar, juice is high in calories, because it takes a lot of fruit to make one small glass. It also lacks the fiber that whole fruit contains, to slow down absorption and prevent Pop Flies.

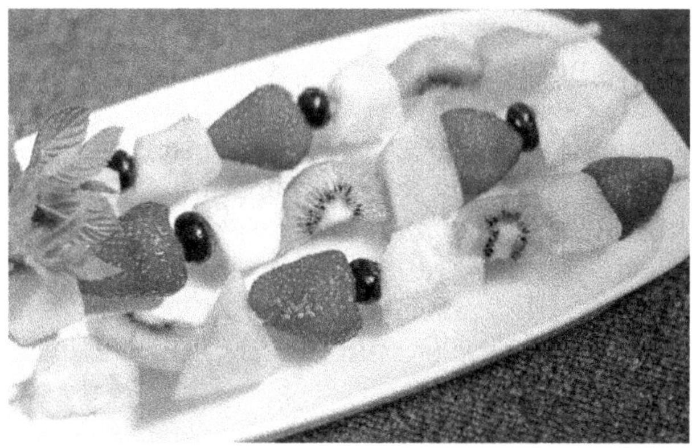

Fruit kabobs are super nutritious and delicious plus they're fun to make and eat. (They also look amazing.) All you need are skewers and fruit, and you've created a fun activity too.

The Plunder of the Victor

I've been touting that sweets should not be a reward, but this is often difficult to carry through. Should you decide to eat or give your child an occasional treat, the simple old-fashioned rule that said, "If you don't eat your dinner, you don't get dessert," should be reinstated as a mealtime motto.

Even if it was possible to remove all sugar from your child's diet, I hesitate to recommend *total* abstinence because it may cause a pendulum effect. When you withhold something that a person really wants, the pendulum will often swing completely in the opposite direction when the opportunity arises. That's what happened to Willie, and now he owns the Wonka Chocolate Factory. Of course, I'm kidding, but the possibility is still there for a similar, but less extreme outcome.

Another reason why you may consider making *a few* allowances is that your children may feel excluded from their friends' events such as holidays and birthday parties. Let children know that sugary foods are to be eaten in moderation or on special occasions, and then set a sensible limit on how much they can eat.

Total denial of sugar now, may also cause them to gorge or horde it later, when you're not around to see it. It's better to ration out sweet treats *in moderation, on occasion*, after they have eaten well, to prevent this from happening. It also teaches them an acceptable amount to eat *on occasion*. It also may help them learn self-control.

The best way to stop the merry-go-round, or the power struggle, is to keep your children well fed with nutritious foods and reasonably occupied with interesting endeavors. Give them high fiber fruits, veggies, beans and whole grains to eat, along with lean protein, nuts, seeds, eggs, and healthy fats (in moderation) until they're full and satisfied, and then help them find something fun or productive to do.

Eating nutritious food first leaves little room for junk food. It's like putting big rocks in a jar first. When you try to add the smaller stones and pebbles of junk food, there's little room for them. On the contrary, obviously, if you put the inferior stones and pebbles in first, there is less room for the big rocks of nutritious foods.

Eat as healthy as possible throughout the day. That way, if you do allow yourself an occasional indulgence, you will have consumed your important nutrients first, and also lessened the desire and room for faux food.

OPPONENT 2: THE FAT CATS

The Sugar Babes and Fat Cats have a ton of slick tricks and sly moves to trip you up and make you fall. It's your task to study their tactics and then act on what you've learned. You met the Sugar Babes in the previous section, so now let's see how the Fat Cats play.

Sugar is bad for health, but so is too much bad fat. Not all people who are overweight crave and eat sweets, so sugar is not the only road to obesity. Many men, for example, can walk away from soda, candy, and cereal, yet these same guys will make a beeline for greasy burgers and fries, or blue cheese and chicken wings, or beer and thick steaks with collars of fat, sizzling hot off the grill. These fat and alcohol preferences contain more calories, gram for gram, than their carbohydrate cohorts. This is one of the reasons why fat eaters and alcohol drinkers gain weight easily. (This fact will be explained in depth in a few more pages.)

Gaining and losing weight is a mystery to some people because they don't know how to play the game. In any sport, you must know the rules in order to beat your opponent. You must know how the enemy operates in order to know what moves to make. Acquiring knowledge and training your mind and body can help you make the right choices to put the odds in your favor, and overcome the foe.

The first fact to ingrain in your brain is that the Sugar Babes and the Fat Cats are the *most powerful players* on the opposing teams. They win over kids and adults by attraction and then beat them by making them weak and obese. These guys are tough to defeat, so expect a lot of opposition when you go up against them.

THE SKINNY ON FAT

Too much of *any kind of fat* will make a person fat, *but* not all fats are bad for you. In fact, some of them are good for you. Good fats are necessary to survive and thrive, but we need to *avoid* the bad fats for the very same reasons.

Both good and bad fat will do the following:

1. Fats are the building blocks of hormones.

2. Fat is fuel for the body and a great source of energy.

3. Fat provides insulation for the body to keep it warm.

4. Fat provides padding for the body in the form of cushions and curves.

5. Fat gives food its flavor and texture and provides a feeling of fullness.

6. Fat is necessary for insulating and developing the brain and nerve tissues.

7. Fat gives sheen to the hair, moisture to the nails, and lubrication to the skin.

8. Fat transports nutrients and aids in the absorption of Vitamins A, D, E, and K.

Hooray for fat! This all sounds great, but before you order a triple-thick shake, we only need *a very small amount* of fat to reap these benefits. *A very small amount.* We're talking **two tablespoons *or less* per day**. Yikes! Right? I've poured more than that over a salad!

Not only do people eat more than two tablespoons of fat per day, but they're eating the wrong kinds of fat. Saturated fat and trans fat raise LDL cholesterol, which can lead to the formation of harmful plaque and possible clogs inside the arteries.

Vegetable oils (canola and olive oil), oily fish (salmon and sardines), nuts, seeds, olives, avocados, and eggs are the best sources of beneficial fats. Omega-3 fatty acids that are found in salmon and walnuts are especially valuable to health because they nourish the brain and reduce inflammation in the body.

The fats in this superior group do not raise bad cholesterol levels (eggs excluded), but actually raise good cholesterol (HDL) instead. Although these fats provide essential nutrients, they should still be eaten in moderation because of their high calories.

Most bad fats are solid or creamy at room temperature. These are your saturated fats, trans fats or partially hydrogenated oils. Animal products such as meat (beef and pork fat, chicken and turkey skin, sausages, hot dogs, bologna, etc.), and whole-fat dairy products (whole milk, butter, cheese, cream cheese, whipped cream, ice cream, and sour cream) and stick margarines and mayonnaise are the worst offenders. Solid fats are also found in palm, and palm kernel oil, and lard.

Extra-virgin coconut oil boasts a few health benefits (which have not been verified through clinical evidence), but it also contains the highest amount of saturated fat (92%) when compared to all fats. Therefore, like all fats, it should be used sparingly because of the dense amount of calories in small amounts. One tablespoon of coconut oil contains 14 grams of fat, 12 grams of saturated fat (over half the average daily allowance), and nary a drop of fiber, protein, vitamins, or minerals.

Trans fats are usually found in commercial or store-bought baked goods and deep fried foods. Think crispy cookies, crunchy crackers, fluffy donuts, and flakey pie crusts, and you're looking at various forms of bad trans fat.

THE FAT CAT STATS

Infants and babies have no fat restrictions because they need fat to develop their brains and nervous systems, and to ensure adequate weight gain. This is why non-nursing infants and babies are fed formula containing fat during their first year, and then whole milk until they're two-years old. After that time, they should drink 1% or 2% milk.

For all other people, the easiest way to keep tabs on **total fat** is to remember your daily calorie range and then eat less than 30% of your calories from fat. This means that adults who consume 2,000 calories a day should eat less than 600 calories (or less than 60 grams) of total fat per day to stay under their daily allowance. An easy way to figure total fat is to take your number from the following chart and multiply it by three.

Total Calorie Intake	Limit on Saturated Fat Intake
1,600 calories	18 grams or less
2,000 calories	20 grams or less
2,200 calories	24 grams or less
2,500 calories	25 grams or less
2,800 calories	31 grams or less

Aim to consume less than 10% of total calories from saturated fat.

Children and adults should limit their total **saturated fat** intake to 10% (or less) of their calories. If adults aim for 2,000 calories a day, the daily allowance of saturated fat would be less than 200 calories (or 20 grams) of saturated fat.

The American Heart Association ***strongly*** *suggests these numbers be even lower*. If you use the AHA suggestion, knock off 3% more from your total. If the average adult uses these numbers, he or she will be closer to reaching their ideal recommended fat limits, rather than not knowing any numbers and grasping in the dark.

Pay close attention to the *fat* numbers on labels. The following list will shed light on the high calories that are found in common foods. Keep in mind that the average person often eats *two-to-four times more* than some of the serving sizes here. When you do the math and then double, triple or quadruple these numbers, you will understand why it is so easy to gain weight after eating high fat foods. Keep your child's daily fat quota in mind as you read these few examples of *total fat*.

- Oil (1 tablespoon) 14g fat (120 calories)
- Potato chips (15 chips) 10g fat (160 calories)
- Cheddar cheese (1 ounce) 9g fat (114 calories)
- Mayonnaise (1 tablespoon) 10g fat (97 calories)
- Breakfast sausage (3 links) 14g fat (170 calories)
- Hamburger 80% lean (3 ounces) 15g fat (231 calories)
- Butter or margarine (1 tablespoon) 12g fat (102 calories)
- French fries, fast food (1 large order) 24g fat (510 calories)
- Ben & Jerry's Vanilla Toffee Bar Crunch Ice cream (1 cup) 40g fat (600 calories)
- Dunkin Donuts Frozen Caramel Coffee Coolatta (large) 47g fat / 29g saturated fat (990 calories) 32½ teaspoons sugar
- Regal movie theater popcorn (1 large tub) 60g *saturated* fat (1,000 calories). That's three *days'* worth of saturated fat!

These opponents will be mentioned in more depth in the "Play-offs" section, since restaurant foods are more inclined to combine multiple players in extreme amounts, which is a whole different ball game.

DON'T LET TRANS FAT UP TO BAT

Trans fat? Put it back! Trans fat is so detrimental to health that the Food and Drug Administration is taking steps to ban its use. Trans fat not only raises bad cholesterol, but also lowers good cholesterol and increases inflammation in the body. The waxy substance also acts like a barrier to prevent healthy nutrients from being absorbed into the body.

Even though food producers are conforming to stricter regulations, trans fat is still found in many cookies, cakes, crackers, pies, frozen pizzas, refrigerated rolls and cookie dough. It is also found in microwave popcorn, donuts, coffee creamers, stick margarine, ready-to-use frostings, pot pies, pancake mixes, and some fast-food French fries (and many other foods that are breaded or battered and deep-fried).

Many products contain trans fat, but don't list it on the label. They are allowed to do so because each serving contains less than 0.5g of trans fat. Yet, if you do the math and calculate what people *really* eat when the serving sizes are multiplied, you up the ante and unwittingly consume trans fat.

So how do you know if trans fat is in the food you eat? Look for words like "hydrogenated" or "partially hydrogenated oils" on food labels. These are trans fat in designer clothes, hoping you won't recognize them with their fancier names. Do not eat trans fat, ever! Avoid it like the plague. Eating a lot of saturated fat, *especially trans fat,* is like pouring grease down the drain and then wondering why the pipes are clogged and the sink is overflowing.

THE GRAND SLAM: ALL WOOD IS NOT CREATED EQUAL

The food that you eat can be compared to wood, and your metabolism is like a fire that is constantly burning calories to keep you alive, energetic, and functioning. The following chart shows that *food grams,* like wood, are not created equal in compactness. There are three different densities that burn at different speeds, even though they are equal in volume.

Carbohydrates and proteins contain 4 calories per gram. Alcohol contains 7 calories per gram, and fat contains 9 calories per gram. Each square is equal in size to symbolically represent one gram, but its density is different because of the calories packed inside. Understanding this concept is one of the keys to making better food choices, and understanding why we gain, maintain, or lose weight.

If you imagine these three gram models as blocks of wood, you can see how fast or slow they'll burn. Protein and carbohydrates are like pine, which burns quickly, because it is a soft wood. Alcohol and fat are like oak, a hardwood, which takes longer to burn because of their density, or concentration of calories.

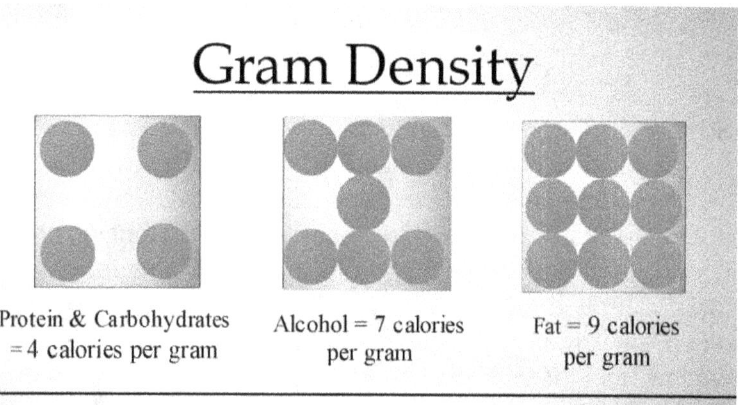

As you can see, alcohol is *almost* twice as dense, and fat grams are *over* twice as dense, as protein and carbohydrate grams, Fat and alcohol contain *more calories in smaller amounts* than complex carbohydrates in larger amounts.

To get a visual of how these concentrated calories stack up, imagine five Buffalo chicken wing drumsticks (mostly fat at 367 calories), next to 3 cups of assorted vegetables and fruit, a slice of whole grain bread, and 4 ounces of grilled skinless chicken breast (super nutritious at 367 calories). The *volume* of food would differ *greatly*, but the calories would be the same. The sad fact is that for all of those chicken wing calories, there is very little meat on them. Most of the calories come from the skin, deep-frying, and the butter-based hot sauce.

The numbers climb on the bathroom scale when too many calories, *no matter what their source,* are consumed before the body can burn off the excess (although the culprits are usually fat, sugar, or alcohol). Since we only needs a specific number of calories per day to survive, the extras are then stored as fat.

To lose fat you must do one, but ideally two things. One is to eat fewer calories in order to force your body to draw from, and burn off, its own storehouse of fat. The second is to stoke your internal flame by adding oxygen to your metabolic fire by-way-of strenuous exercise.

The mere state of being alive burns calories, but being physically active burns even more calories. Aerobic (a term coined in the 1970s that means "with oxygen"), cardio, cardiovascular, or cardiorespiratory are terms used to define exercises that get your heart rate up and pumping to improve oxygen use in the body, which starts the fat-burning, muscle-building process.

Any exercise, activity, or sport that exerts the arms and / or the legs in a continuous motion, stokes the metabolic furnace and fans the internal flame to burn more calories faster. Oxygen sucked into the lungs by way of deep breathing during vigorous exercise cranks up the internal heat and melts fat like butter in a pan.

To get a better picture of this log burning process, imagine a steady flow of oxygen blowing into a campfire. The air forces the flame to blaze higher and the logs to burn faster. Too little oxygen, such as that in a sedentary lifestyle, and the fire smolders low.

Too much air, such as a beginner ramping up a workout, and the fire flares up, but quickly dies down, because the ability to continue at this intensity becomes next to physically impossible for someone who is starting out. The flame of inspiration and the fire of desire are also inclined to fizzle because of the unrealistic intensity.

So how does one create this fat-burning inferno? The same way you build a real campfire. Kindling or softwood always burns first to get the fire started. Your immediate storehouse of carbohydrates is the softwood that burns until the fat logs catch on fire. Once the softwood (carbs) is used up, after about 20 minutes of moderate exercise, activity, or action-packed play, the fire begins to depend on the stored hardwood (fat) as fuel, which begins the fat melting process. It's the twenty to sixty or more minutes of continuous exertion that melts the calories from fat and tones and trims the body.

You can also vary your exercise routine by kicking it up a notch, if you are accustomed to some rigorous activity. When a high intensity is maintained, such as in aerobic interval training, calories will burn faster because the fire is more intense. Walk ten minutes, jog a few minutes, run a few seconds, and then start all over again for one or two sets. As you build up endurance, work toward thirty or more minutes.

Forty-five minutes of vigorous exercise offers the same weight-loss benefits as sixty minutes of moderate exercise. Always consult your physician before beginning any new or intense exercise program.

A few aerobic workouts that you may want to try are walking, biking, skipping rope, swimming in a pool, or hopping on a stepper or rebounder. You may also want to try hula hooping. Thirty minutes of hooping provides the same cardio benefit as walking 3.5 mph on the treadmill. Professional diameter and weight hoops are easy to use and can be twirled almost anywhere. Hula hooping is not only fun and a great workout, but it's also a great way to whittle your waist. You can also lift small weights or do squats or push-ups to add strength training to your regimen. Every minute you workout is like money in the bank. It all counts in the end.

If you don't have time for a complete cardio workout, ten minutes in the morning, ten at noon, and ten at night will improve heart and lung function and provide a happier feeling of well-being.

HOW TO BEAT THE FAT CATS

Now that you know how the Fat Cats play and you understand the rules, this is how you win the game: To lose weight and build muscle, you must eat more complex carbohydrates, lean protein and good fat, and eat less sugar, white flour, and bad fat. Keep your metabolic fires burning by doing any of the aforementioned activities or any other sports that requires exertion for *at least* thirty-to-sixty minutes a day, *most days of the week.* You can break this time up like some experts say, and it will benefit your health, but if you want to melt fat at a faster rate, you must exercise or play at a steady pace as instructed above. Here are a few more ways to beat the Fat Cats.

- ✓ Use ground turkey in place of ground beef.
- ✓ Beware of "healthy" organic food that is still high in fat.
- ✓ Pack a healthy lunch and brown bag it to school or work.
- ✓ Eat smaller amounts of bad fat foods. A LOT smaller amounts.
- ✓ Choose lean cuts of meats (no skin) and low-fat dairy products.
- ✓ Eat low-fat protein and high fiber foods to keep you feeling full longer.
- ✓ Beware of labels that boast, "No cholesterol," but still contain a lot of fat.
- ✓ Beware of labels that flaunt, "No Trans Fat," but still contain a lot of other fat.
- ✓ Add beans or mushrooms as meat extenders in recipes, to use less animal products.
- ✓ Prepare breakfast options ahead of time, so you don't grab inferior foods or skip this important meal.
- ✓ Don't let yourself to get too hungry or you will go into survival mode, crave fatty foods, and then eat like you're starving.
- ✓ Remember your fat limits and then read labels, so you're able to keep score. Do a quick estimate of the fat content before you buy or eat anything.

- ✓ Treat bacon or chicken wings or other such foods as appetizers, not main courses. Make do with one or two of them, if you must indulge.

- ✓ Grill, roast, or broil meat on a rack to keep fat drippings away from the meat as it cooks. (Gravy made from meat drippings should be eaten in moderation.)

- ✓ Take a small plastic bag of nuts, seeds, raisins, baby carrots, or fruit with you when you go out, so you won't be tempted to stop for fast food if you're hungry.

- ✓ Eat healthy fats such as avocados, olive oil, canola oil, flaxseed oil, nuts, seeds, and eggs in moderation to get essential fatty acids and to keep hunger away.

- ✓ Never go grocery shopping when you're hungry and always follow an itemized list. If you are hungry and "listless" in the store, you're more likely to buy inferior food on impulse, especially sugar and fat-laden foods.

- ✓ Don't keep high fat foods in the house where you may be more inclined to eat them. If you must indulge, make the food difficult to reach. For instance, rather than buying ice cream and keeping it in the freezer, go out for a small ice cream cone at the local parlor. Oftentimes, the food loses its appeal because of the effort involved to get it.

Ask yourself, "If not now, when will I start?" When you look back on your life five years from now, will you see progress or that you're stuck in the same place? Even slight movement in the right direction is growth. I used to tell myself, "If I don't do it now, it won't get done. I will always have to go through this difficult place to get where I want to go." Making positive lifestyle choices will never get easier than where you are now. Ready? You're up!

OPPONENT 3: THE SALTY DOGS

"Please pass the salt." How often do we make this request? Whether we lightly sprinkle or liberally shake, too much salt is bad for our health. Yet, we need a small amount of salt to survive. Sodium (salt) works with potassium to perform a watery-balancing act in our cells. Our heart rhythms, nerve impulse communications, and muscle contractions and relaxations all depend on sodium to keep things humming smoothly.

The largest salt mines are found in grocery stores and restaurants where processed and prepared foods line the shelves, coolers, and freezers, and where servers hand it out on lovely dishes or in disposable wrappers to go. Salty Dogs are hidden in everyday foods that most people rarely think about: The boxed and frozen premade meals, the snacks and chips, the canned soups and vegetables, condiments like ketchup, soy sauce, and barbeque sauce, all of which add an ocean of sodium to our daily diets.

The proof is on the label if we take the time to read it, but even then, most people don't know what the numbers mean. So here they are in black-and-white: The average adult should limit their sodium intake to 2,300 milligrams per day. Children should have between 1,000 and 1,300 milligrams of sodium per day.

The American Heart Association recommends that this number be closer to 1,500 milligrams per day for adults. Not only for those who are 51 years or older, for those who are African American, or for those who have kidney disease, high-blood pressure, or diabetes, but for *all* adults. This is just under ¾ of a teaspoon per day. Most people get their daily requirement (and then some) in the foods they eat, without adding more to it.

KEEP PASSING ON THE SALT

The major reason why too much salt is detrimental to health is that it causes the body to retain fluid, which in turn increases blood pressure. When there is an abundance of salt in the diet, the sodium attracts and pulls water into the bloodstream. This increase in blood volume puts added strain on the arteries, which can elevate blood-pressure. Hypertension makes the heart work harder, which in turn damages blood vessels and organs and raises the risk of heart failure, disease, and stroke.

According to government dietary guidelines, 36% of American adults have pre-hypertension, and 34% of them already have hypertension. That's 70% of the population! Almost two-thirds of the United States has, or is on the path to having, high-blood pressure, if they don't make lifestyle changes.

Most people believe that this is a concern for the middle-aged and the elderly, but recent studies have found that 97% of children eat too much salt. This puts them at risk for many of the adult sodium related diseases too. Add obesity to the mix and the risks are even higher. Poor lifestyle habits such as too much faux food and too little physical activity are showing up as high-blood pressure numbers on pediatric charts.

The cause of this quandary is not only faux food and lack of activity, but also commercially processed and pre-packaged foods that often *appear* to be healthy. Salty Dogs are being fed to little tots, as unsuspecting parents assume that what they're giving them is good for them, when it's really not.

The Centers for Disease Control found that three-fourths of baby and toddler foods contain way too much salt for those ages.

Another reason why too much salt is bad, is that it can take you on a bloat ride to a place called *Edema*. Symptoms of edema (water retention) may include muscle aches and pains, shortness of breath and puffiness around the eyes and face. Too much salt may also lead to dehydration.

WHERE DO THE SALTY DOGS ROMP?

Sodium is found in small amounts in healthy foods such as vegetables, dairy products, meat, and shellfish. Though minimal in amount, the numbers quickly add up when combined with other sodium-soaked foods.

As you read the following list, remember the limit of 1,000 to 1,300 milligrams of sodium for children and 2,300 for adults per day. Tally up the foods they eat every day and compare the numbers to their daily sodium quota. The following information is adapted from www.supertracker.usda.gov (foodapedia) or taken directly from the food label. Brands may vary in sodium content.

- Spam (½" thick slice) 758 mg
- Soy sauce (1 tablespoon) 902 mg
- Dill pickle (1 medium) 569 mg
- Banquet Beef Pot Pie (1) 704 mg
- Rice-a-roni (1 cup cooked) 780 mg
- V8 Vegetable Juice (1 cup) 653 mg
- Chicken nuggets (5 nuggets) 446 mg
- Tomato soup (1 cup, canned) 695 mg

- Teriyaki sauce (1 tablespoon) 611 mg
- Cheese-filled Combos (1 cup) 1107 mg
- Olives, stuffed green (5 medium) 269 mg
- Spaghetti sauce with meat (1 cup) 978 mg
- Kraft Macaroni and Cheese (1 cup) 786 mg
- Pop Secret microwave popcorn (1 bag) 890 mg
- Hot dog (with bun and condiments) 920 mg
- Cream of celery soup (1 cup, canned) 1,300 mg
- Ramen noodle soup (3 ounce package) 1,541 mg
- Pizza with cheese and pepperoni (1 slice) 575 mg
- Banquet Salisbury Steak frozen meal (1) 2363 mg
- Chunky chicken noodle soup (1 cup, canned) 823 mg
- Tyson Buffalo Style Chicken Strips (3 ounces) 1040 mg
- Bacon cheeseburger (fast food, 1/4 lb. meat, mayo, and ketchup on bun) 1,655 mg

Even though some of these numbers are alarming, there are many more foods that contain loads of sodium, besides the ones listed above. For example, even though cheese is high in calcium, which is good for you, it's also high in salt and fat so it should be eaten in moderation.

One of the most dangerous traits the Salty Dogs possess is that they're often not perceived as a threat. I suppose that's because the damage they do isn't noticed until it's late in the game. I also suppose that's why hypertension is called "The Silent Killer." Just because you can't see something, doesn't mean that it's not there.

HOW TO SHAKE THE SALTY DOGS

So what can you do about it? Know your numbers and then read labels to make wise food choices.

- ✓ Eat more fruits and veggies. They not only replace the salty foods and snacks, but they also contain potassium which helps minimize water retention by counterbalancing the harmful effects of sodium. The best sources of potassium are tomatoes, potatoes with skin, sweet potatoes, broccoli, spinach, citrus fruits, cantaloupe, bananas, beans, low-fat milk, and yogurt.

- ✓ Use herbs, salt-free spices, citrus juices, and Mrs. Dash Seasoning Blend instead of salt when flavoring food.

- ✓ Select products with low sodium numbers or those that tout 25% or 50% less sodium, or "lightly salted," or "no sodium" on the label.

- ✓ Drink your daily quota of water to flush excess salt from your system. (Divide your ideal weight in half to determine how many ounces you should drink every day.)

- ✓ Read the book *Eat less Salt: An Easy Action Plan for Finding and Reducing the Sodium Hidden in Your Diet with 60 Heart-Healthy Recipes* by The American Heart Association.

When people become accustomed to eating low-salt foods, they are later amazed at how salty the previous "normal" (salted) food tastes, if they eat it.

OPPONENT 4: THE GOOEY GUYS

The Gooey Guys are refined white flour foods and refined white rice. They're on the opposing team, not because of what they possess that's bad, but because of what they *don't possess* that's good. These guys lack fiber and other health building nutrients *that they once did possess,* to keep the body strong and the blood sugar steady, but they now contain little to none of them.

This is because the Gooey Guy manufacturers take a perfect grain of wheat or rice, strip it of its outer covering (the bran that contains fiber, B vitamins, and trace minerals), and then extract the heart of the grain (the nutrient rich germ that contains antioxidants, Vitamins B and E, and healthy fats). What you have left is the pretty white starchy part (the endosperm that is a simple carbohydrate) to make fluffy white rice or doughy white rolls, breads, biscuits, pastries, pancakes, pastas, and many other white flour based foods.

After the refining process removes the fiber, vitamins, and minerals from the grain, the producers toss a few miniscule nutrients into the mix, so they can label their flour or rice "enriched." That way it *appears* to be nutritious when it's really not that great.

Why would they do this? Because white flour makes green money. It's always about sales and cash. Removing the outer coat and germ in a grain of wheat prevents rancidity and limits bug infestation, therefore extending the shelf life. Whole wheat flour stores well for 1-3 months. Refined white flour stores well for 6-8 months. Those five months can make or break a company that's storing and selling flour. Therefore, they opt for the product with the longer shelf-life.

WHY ARE GOOEY GUYS SO BAD?

Once the important part of the grain is gone, the gooey guys are equivalent to eating enriched paste, because there is no substance left in them. In fact, you can make paste with white flour and water. It's true. Google it and see. Even so, since fiber is a ticket to stabilizing blood sugar levels and keeping kids feeling full longer, they're going to feel hungry sooner instead, if they eat these gluey, gooey guys.

The Gooey Guys not only lack fiber and nutrients, but they also create Pop Flies and dips because they're easily absorbed and quickly converted to sugar which ends up in the bloodstream. The result? Gooey Guys cause many of the same problems that the Sugar Babes do. Notice the similarities:

1. They both increase the risk of Type 2 diabetes.

2. They both replace nutrient dense foods in the diet.

3. They both increase the risk of high LDL cholesterol.

4. They both contain little substance and empty calories.

5. They both trigger cravings and compulsive overeating that may lead to weight gain.

6. They both create blood sugar spikes and dips that lead to mood swings, lack of energy, and brain fog.

HOW TO WHIP THE GOOEY GUYS

The major players on the Gooey Guys team are white rice, white breads, white flour tortillas, pastas, Ramen noodles, rolls, pancakes, waffles, muffins, cereals, bagels, pastries, pies, cakes, cookies, crackers, and donuts. Pastas are also on the Gooey Guys team, but there are *a few* redeeming qualities in the durum flour. Most are higher in protein than other white flours, and most contain 2 grams of fiber per serving.

Many of the aforementioned white-based foods can be found with all of their parts intact, such as in whole wheat, rye, oat, and pumpernickel breads and brown rice. Whole grain tortillas, pastas, bagels, rolls, pancakes, waffles, muffins, cereals, and crackers are all excellent choices in their complete form.

The Whole Grains Council recommends that consumers look for the whole grain stamp on food labels. They also advise eating three products labeled "100% Whole Grain" OR six products bearing ANY other Whole Grain Stamp, to meet daily requirements.

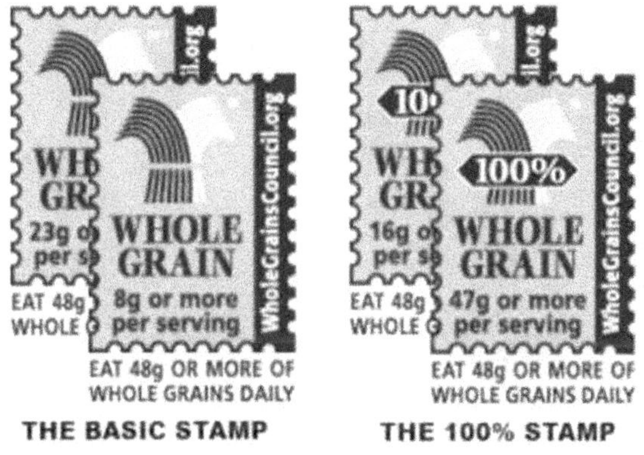

WHOLE GRAIN
8g or more per serving
WholeGrainsCouncil.org
EAT 48g OR MORE OF WHOLE GRAINS DAILY
THE BASIC STAMP
100%
WHOLE GRAIN
47g or more per serving
WholeGrainsCouncil.org
EAT 48g OR MORE OF WHOLE GRAINS DAILY
THE 100% STAMP
Whole grain stamp adapted from wholegrainscouncil.org.

The government nutrition site, choosemyplate.gov, recommends that *at least half your grains be whole grains*. This is a good place to start if you're not used to eating them. Ideally, look for a whole grain listed as the first ingredient on the label or find the whole grain stamp of approval on the package and then eat them instead of a Gooey Guy.

A diet of whole grains reduces the risks of stroke, Type 2 diabetes, heart disease, and weight gain. According to the whole grains council.org, recent studies have found that when whole grains are included in the diet, people experience a reduced risk of colorectal cancer, high blood pressure, tooth loss and gum disease, asthma and other diseases caused by inflammation. Experts have also noticed healthier carotid arteries in those who eat whole grains. I'm all for keeping this pipeline clear, since these arteries supply blood to the brain.

The way to resist a white flour fix is by replacing it with a whole grain food. More on this topic in the upcoming *Fabulous Fiber: Superstar Grains* section.

THE PLAYOFFS

The playoffs are where various teams meet and do their best to win the game. When the Sugar Babes, Fat Cats, Salty Dogs, and Gooey Guys come together in a variety of forms, they're called hyperpalatables, meaning they're very easy to eat. One hit and they tap into the brain's reward system and become addictive to people who are sensitive to these ingredients.

These treacherous foes can swoop up a child and carry him on a trip that leads to obesity and disease. When these hyper-players join forces they often create Olympian-sized, calorie condensed meals that turn innocent opponents into overweight prey. These teams woo children into their happy places and burger palaces with gimmicks and toys, amid gobs of fat, sugar, salt, and starch that send a rush of dopamine, to thrill their budding brains and hook them on a feeling, literally.

The damage these ogres inflict is huge, yet their attraction pulls like the mesmerizing siren song in Homer's *Odyssey*. If left unchecked, these colossal combos can turn a healthy child into an eating machine that gobbles up two-to-three times the calories, he or she would normally eat in one sitting. Studies have shown that when hyperpalatables join forces, it's almost impossible for a person, who craves these foods, to stop eating the meal no matter how large it is, or how full they are, *once they have begun*. The fast food motto seems to be, "No crumb left behind."

One study found that when lab rats were given free rein to eat as much fat, white flour, and sugar-filled foods as they wanted, they nearly ate themselves to death. In this same study, researchers also found that of all the combinations, the sugar-filled foods had the potential to be the most physically addictive like a drug.

Even though a drug feels euphoric to a druggie, you wouldn't feed their addiction by giving them a hit. On the same token, it would be more compassionate to withhold a hyperpalatable meal from a child who has a weakness for these foods.

Adults are not immune to this siren serenade. Hyperpalatables hook full-grown men and women with their addicting appeal, so that all the diseases previously mentioned apply to them too, but with an additional woe thrown in. Experts have discovered that hyperpalatables may be a risk factor for developing Alzheimer's disease. Rats scored significantly worse on memory tests after a 90 day diet of simple carbohydrates and saturated fats. [17] The Sugar Babes, Fat Cats, Salty Dogs, and Gooey Guys strike again!

Although these villains can lure kids in, fast food joints aren't solely to blame. These groups do damage no matter where they play. Here are a few more combinations.

- Foods that contain **sugar and fat** combinations: Ice cream, chocolate, cheesecake.

- Foods that contain **fat and salt** combinations: Potato chips, bacon, cheese, chicken wings, French fries.

- Foods that contain **salt, fat, and refined white flour** combinations: Pizza, cheeseburgers and hotdogs with buns, macaroni-and-cheese, Ramen noodles.
- Foods that contain **refined white flour, sugar, and fat** combinations: Pastries, donuts, pies, cookies, and cakes.

You get the idea. There are many more.

Even if your children aren't hooked on these foods, it doesn't mean these players won't hurt them. Many people aren't addicted to sugar, fat, salt, or refined white products, but because they eat them on a regular basis, they still may gain weight and harm their health.

THE TOP PLAYING FIELDS IN AMERICA

Social overeating and drinking at fast food restaurants are two of the biggest contributors to the obesity epidemic. Millions of people flock to these "playing fields" like pigeons to an old statue. "Let's get a pizza and wings!" "Let's grab a burger and fries!" "Let's go out for ice cream!" This may be fine *on occasion in very small quantities*. I've taken my children to some of these places, on occasion, but when the habit becomes a lifestyle, children and adults gain weight then lose their health and self-esteem.

> *Whoever* holds the
> CAR KEYS and CASH
> chooses the food
> the FAMILY *will eat*

You can see how extreme these hyper-players "play" by visiting each restaurant's website. Check out a meal that you or your child has recently eaten while dining at one of these places, and then look at the calories, saturated fat, salt, sugar, and lack of fiber in each item. Since these numbers only account for *one* meal, and your child may have eaten earlier, or they may be eating and snacking again later in the day, tally the overall count when adding up these shocking numbers to get an accurate picture.

The following is an example of one grilled chicken sandwich combo meal at a fast food restaurant, which you would assume is fairly healthy. The key word in this meal that makes it high in calories and fat is the term *premium*. This doesn't always mean that it's the best. It often means more "stuff" has been added to it during preparation. Using a teenage girl's daily limits, we're looking at 1,800 calories, 60g of total fat, and 2,300mg sodium, and 6 teaspoons of sugar. Her ideal total fiber intake should also be around 25 grams.

One Premium Grilled Chicken Club Sandwich contains 510 calories, 20g of fat, 1,250mg of salt, and 3g of fiber. One medium order of fries contains 340 calories, 16g of fat, 190g salt, and 4g of fiber. One medium cola contains 200 calories, 55g of sugar, and 5g of salt.

The grand total for this meal is 1,050 calories, 36g of fat, 1,445g of salt, 13¾ teaspoons of sugar, and 8g of fiber. Crank these numbers up if your child eats burgers or larger sizes. Add in breakfast, supper and an evening snack or more soda, and your child's numbers will be off the charts for the day.

If you exchanged the cola for a milkshake in the above meal, the numbers across the board would skyrocket. One *medium* chocolate shake topped with swirls of cream and drizzled with syrup contains 700 calories, 97g of sugar (24¼ teaspoons!), and 20g of fat. Bump that up to a large and we're talkin' 850 calories and 30 teaspoons, yes, thirty. Count 'em, 30 teaspoons of sugar in one milkshake! That's *almost* ¾ cup of sugar! And your daughters and sons are supposed to have, what? Six to nine teaspoons of sugar? Yep.

When children fill up on the Sugar Babes, Fat Cats, Salty Dogs, and Gooey Guys, they lose their desire for nutritious foods. Even if they tried to supplement healthy foods with the faux food, they'd be consuming an enormous number of calories to meet their daily nutrient requirements. If you look at the stats, it's easy to see that the bad outweighs any good that could possibly be gleaned from this type of meal. The good news is that when children begin eating real food, their desire for faux food wanes. If they stay away from it long enough and decide to try it again, the meal will often make them feel sick.

This is just one example. Some restaurants and menu choices are slightly better, but many are the same or worse. Now is a good time to pull out that note card with your child's daily limits on it, so you can compare stats. The following websites (search for their name.com) are required by law to post their nutrition information. Take a look and see how much fat, sugar, and salt, and how little fiber the fast food industries are serving your growing children. See the truth, the whole truth, and nothing but the truth, straight from the fast food sources.

1. Arby's
2. Burger King
3. Chick-Fil-A
4. Chuck E. Cheese
5. Domino's Pizza
6. Dunkin' Donuts
7. Jack in the Box

8. KFC
9. McDonalds
10. Pizza Hut
11. Sonic Drive-in
12. Subway
13. Taco Bell
14. Wendy's

The saying is true that "you are what you eat." If you eat good food, you're more prone to feel good and enjoy good health. If you eat bad food, you're more prone to feel bad and reap poor health, but the saying applies to portion sizes too. If a person eats large amounts of inferior food and drinks on a regular basis, it shouldn't be a surprise when that person ends up being large too. Fast food restaurants are notorious for overfeeding people. That's because when serving sizes increase, profits increase. And since most people eat what's in front of them, they feel compelled to finish a meal no matter how large it is, even if they're stuffed.

Lack of activity doesn't lead to obesity. It's the other way around. Obesity leads to a sedentary lifestyle. It's all the high calorie faux food in humongous serving sizes that pack on the pounds and widen the waist, and decrease the desire, ability, and motivation to move. Restaurants are the major playing fields where children congregate to be conquered by gigantic popcorn buckets, triple-decker cheeseburgers, unlimited refills of soft drinks, and jumbo ice cream cones. We'd all do well to limit our visits or stay completely off their turf.

FIRST OUT: KEEP IT FUN!

Limit your fast-food visits to once a month *or less*, or opt for the meal that doesn't offer a toy in the deal. These are the flashy lures that hook people into buying their food for their supposedly "unhappy" children to make them happy. This type of conditioning may eventually teach children to equate unhealthy food with fun or happiness.

If you do choose to take your children to fast food restaurants, help them make better food choices. Select chicken wraps, green salads with low-fat dressing, oatmeal with berries, milk, and 100% fruit juice. But honestly, once you take your children inside, it's difficult to control what they order. Better to stay away altogether or limit eating out or ordering in to once a month, and then wean them away even more over time.

Make your own healthy premade happy meals for the entire family. Prepare grab-and-go foods ahead of time and store them in compartmentalized plastic containers with lids in the fridge. Fill the sections with nuts, grilled chicken strips, cut up veggies and fruit, whole grain crackers, sliced hard-boiled eggs, low-fat cheese, cottage cheese, or unsweetened applesauce for a quick breakfast, a portable lunch, or a snack to go while on the road. The divided containers also help manage portion control.

You can also appease a young child's desire for the faux food and toy by feeding them healthy portable food and then taking him or her to a dollar store instead. The toy is often the big draw of the fast food meal anyway, so give them a couple of bucks and let them get whatever they want: Glow sticks, plastic jewelry, cards, markers, stickers, crayons, coloring or activity books, play money, balls, jump ropes, or sidewalk chalk.

Another alternative to fast food dining is to take the money that you would spend on eating out and buy the ingredients to make unusual or exotic meals or cultural cuisine: Search the internet for Japanese, Chinese, Greek, Mexican, Italian, Polish, Irish, Spanish, Indian, or Polynesian recipes and make the meal a family affair. Let your children help with preparations, add a bit of ethnic décor, and you've also made a memory.

SECOND OUT: KEEP IT CLEAN!

It's difficult to make healthy food and drink choices when we're bombarded by sweet, fatty, salty, gooey foods all day via the media and well-meaning family and friends, but that doesn't mean we should allow these players to control our lives. If your house was infested with bugs and they began showing up everywhere, you wouldn't stop fighting the invasion. How many people would say, "It's just too difficult! Even when I fumigate my home, another colony raids from a different way, so I might as well give up."? No way! We'd do whatever it took to stop them from taking over our lives. We'd caulk every crack and clean every corner to be rid of the pesky pests.

If you think of your children's bodies as the home where their spirits reside, you can see how crazy it would be to let these invaders dominate their lives. A massive faux food infestation adds excess padding to their bottoms and bellies and slowly erodes their health. And even if no outward sign of inward damage were visible, it doesn't mean it's not taking place. The harm from termites often takes place beneath the surface as they chew through supporting joists, and the homeowner lives there unaware until the day the floor caves in and crashes to the ground.

THIRD OUT: KEEP IT NATURAL!

Since the feel good hormone dopamine is one of the key players in the addictive power of hyperpalatables, something must take its place, or the cravings may remain or return. The following are a few natural and healthy ways to raise levels of dopamine and other feel good hormones in the brain. If you eat the following foods and do the following activities, they will help stimulate a natural fix. [18]

1. Eat regularly scheduled nutritious meals to keep blood sugar levels stable.

2. Engage in a bit of friendly competition or vigorous exercise to increase serotonin levels. Exposure to light is also beneficial.

3. Participate in some form of exercise or active play for at least 30 minutes a day. This can be broken up to 10 -10 -10 minutes throughout the day.

4. Spend a few minutes meditating in quiet solitude. Meditation has been proven to raise levels of dopamine and reduce impulsive behaviors.

5. Become more physically active by engaging in fun, challenging, and exciting activities, such as those suggested in the latter half of this book.

6. Become more socially active by engaging in meaningful face-to-face conversations and activities, such as those suggested in the latter half of this book.

7. Set attainable goals for yourself. The desire of a thing, the expectation of a "reward" (reaching your goal), and taking positive steps in the direction of the goal, stimulates the release of dopamine.

8. Participate in a longer more intense workout, or do a series of stretches, or read something funny or watch a comedy. Vigorous activity, stretching, or a genuine belly laugh releases endorphins, a similar mood enhancing and pain-reducing hormone.

9. Eat Omega-3s foods such as salmon, walnuts, chia seeds, and flaxseed; protein rich foods such as skinless chicken, meats, and almonds; an assortment of fresh fruits and veggies, along with whole grain foods, beans, peas, lentils, seeds, and low-fat dairy to create a feeling of well-being. If you choose a wide variety of real, whole food in a rainbow of colors, you'll most likely cover the bases and feel better in general.

The *process of elimination* is indeed a process. Lifestyle changes take time to establish. They also become more deeply ingrained when taken in small consistent steps, rather than vaulted in huge erratic leaps. Radical changes often create rebellious reactions. Firm but steady progress is a key to lasting transformations that become lifelong habits.

The bottom line is it's very difficult for most of us to *completely* give up sugar and junk food. Most people have a tough time resisting sweet treats and fatty foods on birthdays, holidays, or special events, *even when their life depends on it.* If you can do it, more power to you. But for all others, cutting back, tapering off, and then, over-time, limiting or eliminating the day-in-and-day-out avalanche of sugar, fat, and salt, and sugar will lead to better health, a leaner physique, and a happier life.

THE ALL STARS

When people eat junk food for a long time, they often lose the desire for healthy food. When people eat healthy food for a long time, they often lose the desire for junk food. When you begin eating from the All Stars' team, cravings begin to wane for inferior food and drinks. The All Stars also slim down your body and power up your game. Each player is needed to create a dynamic force that can knock out the detrimental habits and effects of being overfed, yet undernourished by the opposing foes.

TEAMMATE 1: FABULOUS FIBER

The most obvious benefit of fiber is that it creates bulk to make elimination easier. Fiber-rich foods also keep heart health in check by whisking wastes and cholesterol away from the intestines and bloodstream. Fiber is also your friend if you want to lose weight and gain health, because high fiber foods take longer to chew and to digest. They also keep blood sugar levels within a healthy range, which keeps you feeling full longer. And the longer you feel full, the less likely you are to overeat and gain weight.

All plant
foods contain FIBER.
NO ANIMAL foods contain FIBER.

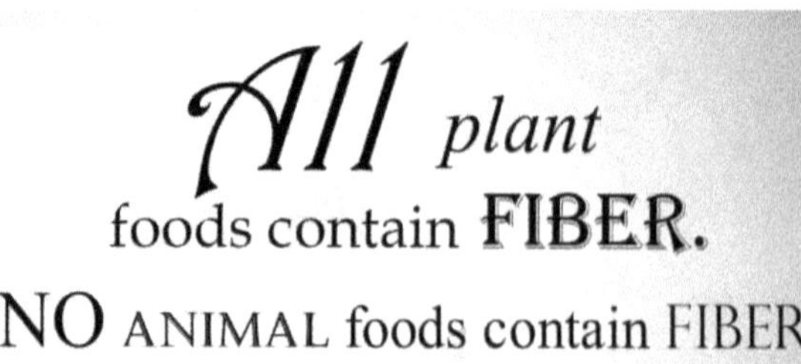

Fiber foods are low in calories and fat (with the exception of avocados, nuts, and seeds), which means there is less chance of becoming overweight, even if you eat a lot of them (as long as fats are not added during preparation or used as condiments).

Therefore, the *majority of the food you eat* should be high in fiber. Choose vegetables, fruits, beans, peas, whole grains, barley, and lentils, along with nuts and seeds in moderation.

Fiber *always* comes from plant sources. If the food has been pulled from the ground or plucked from a stalk, tree, or vine you're good to go, literally. Although all fiber is beneficial to health, apples, oats, peas, beans, and barley are the best sources for lowering cholesterol. Just remember the children's song, "Oats, Peas, Beans, and Barley Grow," and then add apples to the verse.

How Much Fiber Should Children Eat Each Day?

AGE AND GENDER	GRAMS
Boys & girls ages 1–3 yrs	19 g
Boys & girls ages 4–8 yrs	25 g
Girls 9-13 yrs	26 g
Boys 9-13 yrs	31 g
Girls 14-18 yrs	25 g
Boys 14-18 yrs	38 g

The requirements stay the same for 18-50 year old women and men. The numbers then decline to 21 grams of fiber for women and 30 grams of fiber for men.

TEAMMATE 2: SUPERSTAR GRAINS

Whole grains not only contain protein and fiber, but they also contain more vitamins and minerals than their refined white competitors. Look for a whole grain as the first ingredient on the label, and ideally, **3 grams or more** of fiber per serving.

Although the pros and cons of refined white grains versus whole grains were mentioned in the Gooey Guys section, here is a list of foods to look for that lower your risk of diseases and that increase your overall health.

Whole Grains

Bagels	Flatbread	Popcorn
Barley	French toast	Quinoa
Bran	Muffins	Rolls
Brown rice	Oat bread	Rye bread
Buckwheat	Oatmeal	Tortillas
Cereals	Pancakes	Waffles
Cornmeal	Pasta	Wheat bread
Crackers	Pocket bread	Wheat germ
English muffin		Wild rice

Whole grain fiber rich foods absorb water like a sponge, so drink plenty of it to keep things moving through the digestive tract. Fiber plus fluid equals bulk, which keeps you feeling full longer and aids in the process of elimination.

TEAMMATE 3: THE BEST VEGGIE TALES

All vegetables are excellent sources of fiber. They're naturally low in calories and fat and high in vitamins and minerals. Most veggies are loaded with antioxidants and phytonutrients. (*Phyto* in phytonutrients is simply the Greek word meaning *plant*-nutrients.) Antioxidants are defenders of the cells. They zap and neutralize free radicals that age and harm the body.

The benefits of antioxidants and phytonutrients are astounding. Studies have found that they contribute to health and wellness on many levels. Many have already been mentioned. Other benefits may also include the following:

- ✓ They help kill cancer cells.
- ✓ They help detoxify the body.
- ✓ They boost the immune system.
- ✓ They decrease the risk of stroke and heart disease.
- ✓ They decrease the risk of cancer and Type 2 diabetes.
- ✓ They restore DNA damage caused by smoking and the sun.
- ✓ They decrease the risk of age-related macular degeneration.

To glean the greatest health benefits, eat a variety of vegetables in a rainbow of colors. The darker the color the higher the nutrients. Steam, roast, bake, broil, grill, stir-fry, or sauté vegetables to retain their nutrients. (Boiling removes some of the vitamins and minerals.) Eat them raw with low-fat dip, salad dressing, or hummus. Add them to soups, stews, casseroles, and salads. Store salad ingredients in a removable bin in the fridge. That way, everything can be pulled out at once to save on prep time. Prepare a few salads at once and then store them in personal-sized containers for easy access and convenience later. Add ribbon cut spinach or kale to soups, stews or fruit smoothies. Use large lettuce leaves as sandwich wraps.

Avocados are an excellent source of fiber, nutrients, and *good* fat, but because they do contain fat, eat them in moderation.

Vegetables

Asparagus
Beets
Bell peppers
Broccoli
Brussels sprouts
Cabbage
Carrots
Cauliflower
Celery
Corn
Cucumbers
Dark leafy greens
Garlic
Green beans
Green peas
Kale
Lima beans
Mushrooms
Okra
Onions
Peas
Potato (*roasted or baked with skin)*
Pumpkin
Radishes
Red peppers
Red potatoes
Romaine lettuce
Sauerkraut
Spinach
Squash
Sweet potato
Tomatoes
Turnips
Zucchini

Beware of condiment bombs that add empty calories to perfectly good food. Breaded or deep-fried veggies, or those smothered in butter or margarine, drenched in melted cheese, or slathered in sour cream, negate their low-fat benefits. Use plain low-fat yogurt as a sour cream alternative or experiment with spices to make veggie dips.

TEAMMATE 4: THE TRUE FRUIT SNACKS

All fruit, but especially those with edible skins and seeds, contain an abundance of fiber, phytonutrients and antioxidants. Fruit is low in fat, salt, and calories, while high in fiber and nutrients. Neither fruit nor vegetables contain cholesterol.

All of the aforementioned benefits from vegetables also apply to fruit. A few servings of fruit per day may lower the risk of heart disease, stroke, cancers, obesity, Type 2 diabetes, and high-blood pressure.

Fruits

Apples	Grapes	Pears
Apricots	Honeydew	Pineapple
Bananas	Kiwi	Plums
Blackberries	Lemon	Pomegranate
Blueberries	Limes	Prunes
Cantaloupe	Mangos	Raisins
Cherries	Nectarines	Raspberries
Cranberries	Oranges	Strawberries
Figs	Papaya	Tangerines
Grapefruit	Peaches	Watermelon

Cut fruits and veggies into bite-sized pieces and arrange them in a creative way on the child's plate. Children will often eat sliced apples, peaches, or pears, as opposed to chomping into a whole fruit. If fresh fruit is not available or in season, buy frozen fruit to mix in banana smoothies or plain yogurt. Frozen grapes or blueberries also make a refreshing summer treat.

TEAMMATE 5: SUPER LEGUMES

What's a legume, you ask? Why they're those lovely green and yellow peas and multi-colored beans and lentils. Peanuts are included too, but because they're high in fat, they should be eaten in moderation. Legumes are loaded with fiber, protein, vitamins, and minerals, and low in fat. They're among the most nutritious foods on the planet, all to be had for a mere few pennies per serving. If fiber is your friend then legumes are your best friends, if you want to lose even more weight and become even healthier. Aside from breakfast cereals containing bran, the highest amounts of fiber are found in legumes.

Flip through a few cookbooks or search the internet to find recipes that contain as many of these legumes as possible. Look for black, kidney, cannellini, Great Northern, Lima, navy, pinto and soybeans, along with chickpeas, black-eyed peas, green peas and lentils.

As little as one half-cup a day is all it takes to make a difference in your health, although a full cup or more throughout the day is even better, especially if weight loss is your goal. Fill up on fiber foods and legumes often, and excess weight will fall like the Times Square ball on New Year's Eve.

Drain and rinse canned beans before using them in recipes. The following are a few ideas to get you started.

1. Bean soups
2. Baked beans
3. Bean burritos
4. Split pea soup
5. Lentils with pasta
6. Brown rice and beans
7. Beans or peas with pasta
8. Spicy bean dips and spreads
9. Traditional chili or white chili
10. Multi-bean salad with a light dressing

11. Black bean and corn salsa with tortillas
12. Black bean and corn salsa over an omelet
13. Garbanzo or black beans on a tossed salad
14. Beans, peas, or lentils in soups, stews or casseroles

A high fiber diet will keep you feeling full longer, stabilize blood sugar, lower cholesterol, and keep cravings at bay. Supplement ground beef or turkey by adding beans (whole or pureed) to recipes.

TEAMMATE 6: LEAN PROTEIN

Protein is the foundational building block of the body, and it is essential to life. The word protein comes from the Greek word *protos*, which means "the first quality." It is needed first and foremost for all cells, tissues, organs, hormones, and enzymes to function. Protein is also needed to grow bones, cartilage, muscles, blood, skin, hair, and nails.

Protein is broken down in the body on a continual basis, so it needs to be replenished every day to replace and rebuild that which is no longer useful. On the upside of this break-down-build-up cycle, most children and adults in the United States eat enough protein to meet their daily requirement. Many of these same adults actually eat more than they really need every day.

One problem with eating too much protein is that it's usually comes from animal sources, which may contain a lot of dense fat calories that can lead to weight gain. Too much protein is also harmful to those who have kidney problems.

Daily Protein Requirements

2-3 year old children ~ 2 ounce equivalent
4-8 year old children ~ 4 ounce equivalent

9-18 year old girls ~ 5 ounce equivalent

9-13 year old boys ~ 5 ounce equivalent
14-18 year old boys ~ 6 ½ ounce equivalent

This guide is intended for children who get less than 30 minutes a day of moderate physical activity in addition to normal daily activities. Adapted from choosemyplate.gov/food-groups/protein-foods

Choose lean cuts of meat. Remove all fat from beef or pork, and all skin from chicken and turkey. Choose ground turkey or extra-lean ground beef (round or sirloin) in place of ground chuck.

The best sources of animal-based protein:

1. Fish, shellfish, salmon, tuna
2. Lean chicken, turkey, beef, pork, venison
3. Low-fat dairy products
4. Eggs in moderation

The best sources of plant-based protein:

1. Beans, peas, lentils
2. Nuts, nut-butters, seeds
3. Quinoa
4. Tofu

When eating plant-based protein foods, it's best to eat them with one of their counterparts. For example, mingle beans and peas, or nuts and seeds, with whole grains to make a complete protein. New studies have found that eating a complementary food *anytime* within the same day will do the trick to make the necessary food combination work.

The following suggestions do just that. Notice that many of these combinations are the same ones as listed earlier for legumes.

1. Lentils with pasta
2. Brown rice and beans
3. Hummus and pita bread
4. Beans or peas with pasta
5. Bean soup with whole grain bread
6. Peanut butter on whole grain bread
7. Black bean and corn salsa with tortilla chips
8. Traditional chili or white chili with corn bread
9. Black bean and corn salsa omelet with whole grain toast

TEAMMATE 7: NECESSARY DAIRY

Dairy products are essential for the growth and repair of muscles, bones, and teeth. Milk is an excellent source of protein, bone-strengthening calcium, potassium, and Vitamin D. Yogurt is also a protein carbohydrate blend that stabilizes blood sugar. It also contains calcium and acidophilus, those friendly bacteria that eat up bad bacteria like little Pac men in your digestive tract. Be sure to read the label and choose yogurts containing live and active cultures.

Low-fat dairy products provide the same health benefits as their full-fat dairy counterparts, but with less of the unhealthy fat. Some producers add sugar to low-fat dairy to make up for the missing taste, once the fat is removed.

A cup is always a standard cup when measuring serving sizes for milk and yogurt. A cup of cheese *equivalent* is 1 ½ *ounces* of hard cheeses, 1/3 cup of shredded cheese, 2 ounces of American cheese, ½ cup of ricotta cheese, or two cups of cottage cheese.

Daily Recommendation for Dairy

Children

2-3 years old 2 cups

4-8 years old 2½ cups

Boys and Girls

9-18 years old 3 cups

Hard cheeses such as cheddar are higher in fat than soft cheeses like mozzarella. One way to indulge in hard cheese without adding too many fat calories is to shred it, to make it "lighter," and then add it to meals and recipes. Always choose low-fat versions of milk, cheese, and ice cream. Many people would never dream of drinking whole milk, yet these same people think nothing of eating full-fat cheese or full-fat ice cream.

The downside of modern-day dairy: most yogurts contain a lot of sugar, but it's not *all* refined sugar. Plain yogurt has no added sugar, yet a 6-ounce container contains about 12 grams of natural milk sugar in the form of lactose. It's the fruit flavored varieties that jack-up the sugar count when the producers add about 14 grams of refined sugar (3 ½ teaspoons) per 6 ounce container. Therefore, when you see the grand total of 26 grams of sugar per serving of yogurt, it means that slightly more than half of the sugar is added refined sugar. The way around this is to eat plain yogurt with a bit of honey and your own fruit mixed in. If you buy store brands, choose yogurts with the lowest possible grams of sugar per serving.

Most cheeses are high in fat and salt. Try low-fat versions or soft cheeses like feta, mozzarella and parmesan. Swiss cheese is comparatively low in sodium. Shredded cheese lightly sprinkled over food adds a cheesy flavor without all the calories.

Dairy is an animal based food, so it contains no fiber, although Activia and Fiber One yogurts add fiber to their products.

Butter, cream, ice cream, whipped cream, sour cream, and cream cheese contain a great deal of fat and very little calcium. Use in moderation or try these substitutions:

- Olive oil instead of butter
- Plain yogurt instead of sour cream
- Frozen yogurt instead of ice cream
- Greek yogurt or tofu instead of cream cheese

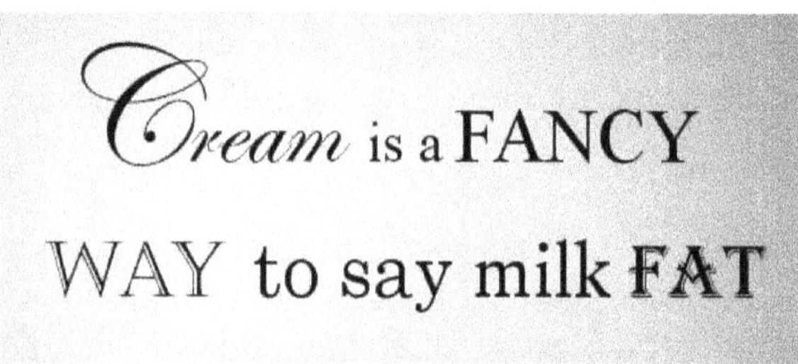

If you substitute the word *fat* for *cream* in dairy product descriptions, you'll get an accurate picture of what you're really eating in these foods: Ice fat, light fat, heavy fat, whipped fat, sour fat, sweet fat, and fat cheese.

TEAMMATE 8: WONDERFUL WATER

You may be tempted to skip this section because you know the importance of water, but do you know the signs of pre-dehydration? People can live for weeks without food and months without certain nutrients before seeing adverse effects, but go a day or two without water and the body begins to shut down.

Life starts getting rough on the throes of dehydration. *Thirst is the first sign that it's knocking at your door.* Many people are mildly dehydrated at any given time, without even knowing it. A lack of water can cause a person to feel tired, listless, or lethargic. Beginning stages of dehydration are dry skin, mouth, and chapped lips. Lack of water may be the cause of constipation, muscle cramps, headaches, extreme fatigue, and irregular blood pressure. Other symptoms include lack of tears, lack of urine (over the course of the day), and dark yellow or orange urine, often accompanied by a strong smell. If the urine is brown get to an emergency room, pronto! Severe dehydration can lead to death.

If you've ever forgotten to water a plant, you've seen the effect it can have on a living thing. When you water it again, the drooping plant often perks up to its lovely succulent self within a matter of hours. We're a lot like that plant, wilted and withered when we haven't drunk enough from this Fountain of Youth. We also see this shriveling effect when luscious plums and grapes are dehydrated into wrinkly prunes and raisins.

Water flows in-and-out of every cell and fiber of our being. It's the source of saliva, tears, bile, urine, and amniotic fluid. The human body is composed of about 60% water that must be replenished daily in order to keep us from dying within a few short days. Water is so important to survival that one mere day in a desert without it and a person is a goner. Three to five days without water is the average max for the average person, under average circumstances, before they teeter on the edge of eternity.

Water is a healing tonic that wipes out many ailments that are often blamed on other causes. The following are a few of the rejuvenating wonders of this crystal liquid.

- ✓ Lubricates the joints.
- ✓ Acts as an appetite suppressant.
- ✓ Aids in digestion and weight loss.
- ✓ Hydrates the skin to make it look supple.
- ✓ Reduces the likelihood of kidney stones.
- ✓ Flushes toxins from the body via the kidneys.
- ✓ Improves energy and physical performance.
- ✓ Energizes the muscles. (Muscles are 73% water.)
- ✓ Transports nutrients to cells and aids in their absorption.
- ✓ Provides a feeling of refreshment and overall well-being.
- ✓ Flushes impurities through the pores and helps the skin stay clear.
- ✓ Moisturizes the air in the nose, throat, and lungs to make breathing easier.
- ✓ Invigorates the brain to make it more alert and efficient. (The brain is 80% water.)
- ✓ Whisks away waste in the large intestines, especially when drunk with fiber rich foods.

- ✓ Regulates body temperature and metabolism through perspiration, respiration, and evaporation.
- ✓ Thins out thick mucus in the lungs and throat to alleviate congestion and breathing difficulties.
- ✓ Keeps blood flowing well. Blood is primarily made of water (85%), and it becomes thick without adequate hydration. Thicker blood makes the heart work harder as it pumps sluggish blood throughout the body.

A child should drink even more fluids, in addition to his daily requirement, to replenish what has been lost due to extenuating circumstances such as those below:

- Any illnesses that involves fever, vomiting or diarrhea. Sip small amounts throughout the day.
- Hot weather with lots of sun and sweat calls for more water. (Extreme heat with hot, flushed skin, but no sweat may be a sign of heatstroke. Seek medical care immediately.) Take bottled water with you when you go out.
- Vigorous play, sports, or exercise that makes a child sweat. (This is another time to watch for signs of heat exhaustion or heat stroke.) Drink water before, during, and after exercise or vigorous activity.
- Indoor heating that dries the air also dries the skin and mucus membranes in the nose, throat, and lungs. Dry orifices allow germs to penetrate the body more easily, where they may possibly cause an illness. Humidify the air and drink more fluids when the air is dry.

Although 20% of our fluids come from food, especially fruits and veggies, the majority of our liquids should come from good old-fashioned water and other healthy water-based fluids, such as 100% fruit juice or low-fat milk or herbal teas. Replace sugary drinks with infused water. Encourage water intake by adding fruit for fun and color. Pretend you're at a fancy restaurant and serve your young customers water from a pitcher or fruit hooked to the rim of the glass. Add blueberries, strawberries, raspberries, or lemon, orange or cucumber slices, along with a sprig of spearmint, and then serve it in a pretty glass or goblet. They'll also be getting a bit of Vitamin C if they eat the fruit too. Give each child a pitcher or flask and then let them create their own refreshing and healthy aqua delight to drink throughout the day.

The easiest way to calculate a child's fluid needs is to cut their weight in half. Therefore, a 128 pound teenager should drink 64 ounces (8 cups) of fluids a day. An additional two cups are recommended, two hours before strenuous exercise, especially in hot weather, and then a half-cup every 20 minutes thereafter while participating in the activity.

Drink an eight ounce glass of water first thing in the morning when you wake up. Drink another full glass about thirty minutes before eating lunch and supper. Three cups down, five more to go. Drinking water before meals also curbs your appetite. You may also want to use refillable water bottles with markings on the sides, to let you know how many ounces you have drunk throughout the day.

One other fascinating fact about water is that hunger is often mistaken for thirst, so reach for a glass of water instead of reaching for food. It just may do the trick and take the edge away.

THE WINNING STRATEGIES

A number of changes in the past forty-plus years have contributed to the obesity epidemic. It's not just the sedentary lifestyle of social networking and electronic gadgets that are completely to blame. A major cultural shift took place back in the 1970s. I'm old enough to remember how things used to be, and this is what I've observed.

Before this time, it was rare to see an obese child or young adult. If you find that hard to imagine, flip through a few pre-1970s photos or history books and you'll become a believer. In the early 20th century up until the 1970s, the average family consisted of a mom who stayed home and took care of the children, and a dad who drove to work in the sole car that they owned. This meant that if you didn't take a bus to school, you usually walked or biked there, or anywhere else that you needed to go.

The average town had one or two diners or family style restaurants. Fast food joints were still in their infancy, and Buffalo wings weren't "invented" yet. (Chicken wings were usually thrown away.) Credit cards were a rarity, which meant that access to extra funds to splurge on dining out was uncommon at this time. An occasional cola at the soda fountain, or a tiny bottle of soda along with a small bag of potato chips (by today's standards) was an infrequent treat.

The average home-cooked meal and restaurant portion sizes were smaller than we see today, and the word supersize was neither heard of, nor used to describe any amount of food. There were no microwaves to heat meals, if someone came home late for supper. There were no premade meals to buy in the frozen food aisle, except TV dinners that needed to heat in the oven for almost an hour. There were no helpers for hamburger. No delis in the supermarkets spinning roasted chickens. No mayonnaise laced salads displayed behind glass cases to take home in a pinch if needed. Nope, moms made almost everything from scratch back then. She even froze or canned fruits and vegetables to store for future use.

Logic dictated that for convenience sake and mom's sanity, there were three square meals a day with no snacks in-between, although they often ate something like fruit, popcorn, or cereal in the evening. The majority of people ate breakfast and supper together as a family and carried lunch boxes of food (that mom had packed) to work or to school. They ate real meat and produce in normal portion sizes, along with a glass of milk. People rarely had second helpings. Sometimes they had dessert, but it wasn't an everyday deal. Sweet treats were doled out in small measures for birthdays and special occasions, a pie, a cake, or a batch of cookies, but even then, people didn't eat dessert until after they had eaten their supper.

As a child my family's **MENU**
consisted of TWO choices:
take it, or leave it.

Buddy Hackett, Comedian

After mom's household duties were done, she sewed or crocheted or attended the community quilting bee, or some other face-to-face function. She often strolled her toddlers around town, organized the church lawn fête, or went to PTA meetings, all of which sound a bit droll when compared to today's busy clamor of activities.

The difference was that these social interactions built lasting friendships that gave her a sense of purpose and meaning in life. Ironically, most of the activities didn't use food to entice new members to their meeting, or keep the existing ones there. Sure, there were parties and potlucks and coffee klatches with coffeecakes, but they weren't like some events today where the big draw is often a table piled high with sticky, fatty, gooey guys from the opposing teams.

The era of *I Love Lucy, Leave it to Beaver,* and *Ozzie and Harriet* was coming to a close and a new age was dawning, so that by the time the 1970s rolled in, birth control had become widely available and wildly popular, and life as they knew it began to change. The women's rights movement burst onto the scene with brassieres ablaze. More women began attending colleges and working outside the home. Mom's second income meant a second car, which meant less walking or biking for everyone.

Fewer children in the family meant extra cash to stash, or to splurge on timesavers like ordering-in or eating-out. Fast food restaurants began popping up like mushrooms in a dank field, and soon became a welcome reprieve for the harried and hurried wife and mother. Especially since most dads at that time didn't believe in doing the cooking.

Fast forward forty years to an average family today: Mom's still bringing home the bacon too, but someone else is metaphorically frying it. That's because mom and dad are often too tired, or too caught up in a time crunch to whip up a home-cooked meal. With fewer children in the family and more money and plastic in our pockets, it's easier to go out-to-eat, or order-in. It's simple to throw a pizza in the oven, or zap a meal in the microwave, or buy frozen or dehydrated dinners, than to slave over a hot stove. Premade meals and restaurant food often trump home-cooking due to the sheer volume of responsibilities and lack of time or energy on the parents part. Therefore, choices are often made and based simply on convenience to make life easier. Not only that, but kids often dictate the menu, and since mom and pop are too pooped to cook, they often grant their requests.

So what's a parent to do? We'll never return to the simple days and ways of our ancestors, but we can reinstate some of the good habits that they had back then. It's true that most kids like faux food, but it's also a fact that they like good food too, if you offer it to them *first* and don't back down when they vote for the opposing teams. You are still in charge, coach. If they refuse to eat good food, so be it. Let them go hungry for a couple of hours. They won't starve in that amount of time. Don't focus on their resistant behavior. Tend to your business and keep the attitude of "this is the way it is now." When hunger strikes hard enough a child will eat healthy food and actually enjoy it.

To reap the benefits of excellent health and to maintain an ideal weight, we must imitate the four positive habits that our predecessors had in their lives.

1. **They ate food that was close to its natural state.**

2. **They had regular mealtimes and ate healthy snacks.**

3. **They ate normal portion sizes.**

4. **They were physically active and socially interactive on a face-to-face basis.**

So without further ado, I present to you, the top four things that our ancestors did right to maintain better health, a lean physique, and a happier life.

STRATEGY 1: THE REAL DEAL

Years ago, people ate food that was close to its natural state. They planted gardens or purchased produce from the farmer's market or shopped for real food at the grocery store. They didn't have much choice in what they ate, because there weren't a lot of choices outside of home-cooked food.

Today, not so much. With the onslaught of advertisers wooing people to their goodies, and so many selections on supermarket shelves and restaurant menus, it's often a hassle to wade through the web of information. It takes time to interpret promotional lingo. And it takes effort to calculate and understand what's really in a product.

So aside from the obvious reading the ingredient label, and eating the whole, real foods, mentioned earlier, there's another way to make quick assessments, and that is to group foods into one of three categories (worst, better, best), and then shoot for the latter two, while allowing for the worst on *rare* occasions. Once you get the idea of how this works, it's easy to rate your food choices. The following are a few examples.

FOOD AND FOOD PREPARATION CHOICES

Worst	Better	Best
Deep-fried	Grilled / Sautéed	Baked / Broiled / Steamed
Pork sausage	Skinless chicken	Fish
Shortening	Canola Oil	Olive oil
Premium Ice cream	Frozen yogurt	Banana fruit smoothie
Cream-based soup	Clear-based soup	Puréed veggie-based soup
Creamy salad dressing	Clear salad dressing	Fruit juice salad dressing
Ground chuck	Ground beef 97% lean	Ground turkey
White rice	Brown rice	Quinoa
Potato chips	Tortilla chips	Popcorn

Most faux foods, most methods of food preparation, and most condiments have similar, but healthier substitutes that can cut hundreds of empty calories from a person's diet. These substitutes can also add more fiber, vitamins, and minerals than those on the opposing team. Cook most of your meals at home from real foods such as fresh produce and whole grains. If you don't know how to cook nutritious meals, ask someone to teach you, or scour the internet for healthy meal ideas and "how-to" videos.

You may not always make the best food choices, but better is healthier than the worst. If you buy junk food the majority of kids will eat it, but it's also true that if you buy fresh, whole, real food, they will eat that too. Even a finicky eater will eat nutritious food if they're hungry enough and they don't have junk food to fall back on. They won't be deprived or feel unloved (maybe upset, but not unloved) if you leave the faux food in the grocery store or restaurant. Over time, when they adjust to the changes, their taste buds and waistlines and even their skin will thank you for it.

STRATEGY 2: THE RIGHT TIME

Years ago, people had structured mealtimes and ate healthy snacks. Structure is good. Without it, buildings fall down and plans fall apart. When regular mealtimes are established, the habit eventually becomes second nature and therefore easier to follow. When there are no set boundaries, eating becomes a hit-and-miss affair, where anything often goes. When this happens, food and eating become the uppermost thoughts in the mind, and when thoughts are consumed with food, people consume food. I discovered this in my own life when I obsessed about food and became a compulsive overeater, gorging or grazing all the day long. I quickly learned that where the mind goes the body follows, as in my frequent rendezvous' where I stumbled bleary-eyed toward the visions of pastries, chocolates, and sundaes swirling through my head.

To rein in thoughts of food and to prevent overeating, meals should ideally be compartmentalized into regular time-slots. Although difficult to do at first, this is one of the best ways to lose weight and to keep it off for good. Once a meal is planned, prepared, and eaten, it is over and done with until the next scheduled time. This way, thoughts of food can be put out of the mind until it's time to prepare the next meal and eat again. (The best time to plan your evening meal is in the morning after breakfast. Meat can be taken out of the freezer to thaw and a quick inventory can be taken to ensure necessary ingredients are on hand.) If weight loss is your goal, be sure to eat enough high-fiber foods and low-fat protein to keep you satisfied until the next meal.

Structured eating should not only be scheduled, but also planned and consistent. The best way to incorporate this routine is to set approximate times for each meal and then strive to eat as close as possible to those times every day. For example, if your mealtime range falls within a twelve hour period, such as 8 AM to 8 PM, you would be eating three-to-four times a day, every three-to-four hours. This pattern is successfully used with slight variations in other structured settings, such as boot camps, boarding schools, and other places of education and training. I used this method myself to control my appetite and to stop binging and compulsive overeating: Three square meals, one snack, nothing in-between.

Strive for this schedule for everyone in the family (except young children), and then fill the in-between eating spaces (when not in school) with fun or productive activities such as those suggested in the latter half of this book. Make every meal a happy meal with lively and fun conversations. Ask your children about their day and then tell them about yours.

Tiny tots and young children have lots of energy and little stomachs so they need more frequent feedings, possibly up to six times a day. A healthy snack between each of the three meals will keep the little ones from becoming too hungry and keep their blood sugar level from falling too low.

Always have nutritious food on hand. This sounds like a no-brainer, but I have often stood gazing in my refrigerator or cupboards, wondering where the healthy food was when there was none to behold. There wasn't any because I didn't buy enough of it to last me through the week. I often have to tell myself, not only to buy nutritious food, but also to stock up on it.

To prevent this from happening, I keep a running grocery list tacked up in a visible place to jot down items when they're getting low. On the following pages I offer a few healthy ideas for each meal, for you to add to your own list.

Breakfast: Start Off on the Right Foot

Adults and children should eat a hearty breakfast because it raises and stabilizes blood sugar after fasting all night. These foods also keep the appetite and emotions happy for a few hours until the next meal. The best breakfast choices are foods of substance such as low-fat protein and whole grain fiber, nuts, seeds, or eggs in moderation. Studies have proven that those who eat a healthy breakfast lose weight easier, keep it off longer, and have more sustained energy throughout the day.

Dairy – Milk, yogurt, and cheese are obvious choices of low-fat dairy. Buy plain yogurt and sweeten it with raw honey or real maple syrup and real fruit. Make yogurt parfaits in fancy glasses layered with fruits and topped with nuts. Whip up a yogurt fruit smoothie in the blender. Try a small bowl of cottage cheese topped with fruit.

Grains – Use whole grain breads for toast with peanut butter or 100% fruit spreads or honey. Try whole grain French toast, waffles, or pancakes topped with fruit or a drizzle of pure maple syrup. Add blueberries and sunflower seeds or sliced bananas and walnuts to pancakes before flipping them on the griddle.

Try whole grain English muffins or bagels topped with eggs and cheese or peanut butter and fruit. Bake whole grain muffins with nuts, berries, raisins, or shredded apples or carrots.

Eat whole grain cold cereals, oatmeal, Whole Grain Cream of Wheat, homemade granola, and Muesli (refrigerator oatmeal). Add sliced bananas or berries to cereal or sprinkle on nuts or sunflower seeds for additional fiber, protein, and nutrients. Search the internet for recipes to make your own healthy breakfast bars, power cookies, or high fiber muffins.

Prepare muffins and freeze them for a portable power-packed breakfast to go. Take them out a few hours before eating or pop them in the microwave for thirty-seconds to thaw.

Protein – Protein foods that pack a punch are lean ham and eggs, peanut butter on whole grain bread or apple slices, and any of the aforementioned whole grain foods with added nuts or seeds, all of which make a complete protein.

Fruit – All fresh, frozen, canned, or dried fruit fall into this group: Apples, bananas, cherries, grapes, grapefruit, oranges, blueberries, blackberries, raspberries, strawberries, kiwi, cantaloupe, honeydew, watermelon, mangoes, peaches, pears, plums, pineapple, nectarines, tangerines, and 100% fruit juice. Buy unsulfured dried fruit such as dates, figs, apricots, raisins, and prunes or dehydrate your own fruit. Add spinach or kale to fruit smoothies. Sprinkle in flaxseeds or chia seeds for added protein, fiber and healthy fats.

NOTE: If you use a juicer or peel the edible skin from fruit, most of the fiber and some of the nutrients are lost.

Lunch & Dinner: Energy throughout the Day

Dairy – Serving suggestions are the same as above. You may also try making a batch of brown rice pudding with low-fat milk or grilled cheese sandwiches on whole grain breads. Sprinkle shredded cheese over soups, stews, eggs, pasta, casseroles and vegetables for added flavor and calcium.

Protein – Sources of animal protein are fish, seafood, shellfish, skinless chicken, turkey, ground turkey, venison, lean beef, ground round or sirloin, pork, and lamb. Try beef or bean tacos, white chili with chicken, scalloped potatoes (with skins) and ham, egg salad sandwiches on whole grain bread, grilled tuna and cheese on whole grain bread, turkey sandwiches with loads of veggies, chicken salad with low-fat mayo, chili and cornbread, chicken wraps stuffed with veggies, or turkey sausage or turkey burgers on whole grain buns.

Experiment with sandwiches and wraps. Combine tuna, diced chicken, or turkey with low-fat mayo or plain yogurt and then add a few spices to the mix. Toss in a few chopped grapes and sunflower seeds or chopped apples and walnuts. Layer sandwiches with sliced avocados, red peppers, or red onions. Mix it up with shredded carrots, cabbage, cucumbers, or spinach leaves.

The best sources of plant protein are beans, peas, and lentils of every shape, size, and color. Add these legumes liberally to soups, stews, casseroles, and salads. Protein is also found in nuts, nut butters, and seeds of every kind such as almonds, cashews, chia seeds, flaxseed, hazelnuts, peanuts, pecans, pistachio nuts, pumpkin seeds, sesame seeds, sunflower seeds, and walnuts.

Make your own healthy mix of slivered almonds or walnuts, sunflower, pumpkin, chia, or flax seeds, and coconut flakes to sprinkle on yogurt, cereal, green salads, fruit salads, and stir-fries. Blend natural peanut butter and raw honey together to use as a protein-rich dip for apples, carrots, celery, and whole grain pretzels. Nuts and seeds are excellent sources of fiber, protein, and healthy fats, but they should be eaten in moderation because they are high in calories.

Vegetables – The brighter the color the more nutritious the food. Choose colorful veggies such as beets, carrots, dark lettuces, yams, tomatoes, red, green, and yellow peppers, spinach, broccoli, kale, cabbage, celery, red potatoes, squash, avocados, Brussels sprouts, cucumbers, corn, red onions, and garlic.

An easy way to add more veggies to your diet is to experiment with different types of salads, such as Mexican Fiesta, Greek, Mandarin, and Caesar. Add strips of grilled chicken, lean steak, or shredded cheese to a plate of mixed veggies and dark greens to make a meal. Toss in garbanzo beans and a sprinkle of sunflower seeds for added protein and fiber. Add grapes, orange slices or diced apples and a few walnuts to a baby spinach salad for a sweet variation. Drizzle a light dressing over the top then add herbs to enhance the flavor. Top a summer salad with blueberries, sliced strawberries, and slivered almonds for a refreshing light meal.

Another way to add more vegetables and whole grains to your diet is by eating veggie pizzas, veggie subs, or veggie wraps. Add extra vegetables to soups, stews, and casseroles. Stuff pocket breads and wraps with assorted veggies such as spinach, shredded carrots, cucumbers, tomatoes, red onion, red peppers, or black olives. Pile turkey sandwiches high with assorted veggies on whole grain bread. Add a cup of vegetable soup for a super nutritious meal.

Fruit – The same suggestions apply here as mentioned above for breakfast. Make a colorful fruit salad and top it with a dollop of plain yogurt mixed with raw honey and a few chopped walnuts. Let your children make their own fruit kabobs. Add thin slices of bananas, apples, or strawberries to peanut butter sandwiches or wraps. Keep fruit in a bowl on the kitchen counter where your children will be more apt to see it and eat it.

Grains – Again, same as above for breakfast, but with a few variations for later meals. Eat whole grain rolls, pocket breads, flat-breads, tortilla shells, English muffins, bagels, brown rice, wild rice, barley, quinoa, whole grain crackers, and popcorn are all excellent choices.

A time-saving tip for evening meals is to use a slow cooker. Prepare meals the night before and then store them in the fridge. In the morning take the crockpot out, plug it in, and set the timer. When you come home from work, serve the meal with sliced bread and a tossed salad, and you have a full course meal. Most foods that are simmered or baked can be cooked in a slow-cooker, such as stew, chicken, chili, meatloaf, or scalloped potatoes and ham.

Another time-saving tip is to cook lean ground beef or chicken breast strips in bulk and then divvy them up into meal-sized containers and freeze. Add the meat to soups, a stir-fry, or casseroles for a quick meal.

Snacks at Home: Kid Approved

Keep healthy snacks in a special pull out bin or at eye-level in the fridge. Cut a variety of fresh produce and make mixed snack bags or containers to grab-and-go. Veggies may include mini-cucumbers, radishes, grape tomatoes, peppers, celery, raw cauliflower, and broccoli. Fresh fruits may include grapes, orange segments, cherries, blueberries, blackberries, red raspberries, strawberries, or cubed pineapple, cantaloupe, honeydew, and watermelon.

Produce sections in grocery stores now offer individual veggie or fruit cups and premade fruit and veggie trays. Although a bit pricey, they are healthy alternatives in a pinch, or while on a road trip, or if your child takes a lunch to school. Scour the produce aisle. Learn your way around the place to know what is available. The following are a few more quick and easy food ideas to serve as snacks or as part of lunch.

- ✓ Deviled eggs
- ✓ Hot-air popped corn

- ✓ Pita chips with hummus dip
- ✓ Frozen 100% fruit juice bars
- ✓ Whole grain crackers with cheese
- ✓ Tortilla chips with salsa or bean dip
- ✓ Frozen banana and berry fruit smoothies
- ✓ Apple slices with cheese or peanut butter
- ✓ Guacamole with whole grain tortilla chips
- ✓ Whole grain cereal with berries or sliced bananas
- ✓ Pretzels dipped in honey mustard or peanut butter
- ✓ Peanut butter and banana slices on mini-pretzels
- ✓ Mini-pizzas with grilled chicken or turkey pepperoni on whole grain English Muffins or pocket bread

For a group of children, arrange an assortment of snacks on a Lazy Susan or a similar tray. Place cut up fruit in one section and cut up veggies in another. Place a few nuts, cheeses, and whole grain crackers in the other sections and then give it a whirl. Skewer cheese and grapes with colored toothpicks or pretzel sticks, to make eating nutritious food fun for them.

NOTE: When doling out snacks, place one serving from the package into a bowl and then put the rest away. Never eat food straight from the bag or box. Studies have shown that the bigger the package the more kids will consume when eating directly from it.

Snacks to Go: You Can Take Them With You!

One of the easiest ways to stave off starvation or thwart temptation while out-and-about is to take something with you to eat. This sounds like it goes against the grain of scheduled meals, but it really doesn't if you make it one of your snacks or mini-meals. The idea is to have healthy food with you if you're going to be out for more than a few hours. Better to carry portable food to keep hunger under control when going on short jaunts, than to raid the nearest fast-food joint or ice cream parlor.

Most of these suggestions are the "Best" food choices, but a few of them fall under the "Better" choice list. All of them are better than the "Worst" choices that are found in most restaurants and convenience stores.

Carry a plastic zip-style bag of bite-sized Shredded Wheat, Wheat Thins, Triscuits, raisins, walnuts, almonds, peanuts, or pistachio nuts. Take a mini-cooler or an insulated lunch-bag (with a re-freezable icepack) to hold bottled water, 100% fruit juice, individually wrapped string cheese, sandwiches, and fruits or veggies when headed out on day trips.

When blood sugar drops, people tend to eat foods they normally wouldn't eat (and more of it). It's not always a lack of will-power. It's the body shifting into survival mode. If you carry healthy snacks, you'll be less likely to stop at the aforementioned places or pick up soda, candy, and chips at the nearest convenience store. You'll also save yourself a chunk of change.

STRATEGY 3: THE PRECISE SIZE

The third thing that our ancestors did right is that they ate normal portion sizes. A child and an adult obviously have different calorie needs. A six-foot man and a six-year old girl are not going to eat the same deck of cards-sized meat serving. Most men laugh and say it's too little. Most kids cry and say it's too much. One size does not fit all.

A general rule of thumb in determining the serving size for a small child is to take a look at *his or her* hand. The answer to *your* serving size question is also in *your* hand. A man's portion size? Yup, in *his* hand. Use the child's hand as a guide to give you an approximate measure of how much he or she should be eating per serving. No matter how young or old your children are their hand is their own personal gauge. Using the hand as a guide automatically customizes serving sizes for men, women and children.

This method of measuring food works because of how we are individually made. Each of us has a heart that is proportionally the size of *our own* fist. Our empty stomachs are also proportionally the size of *our own* fist. It stands to reason that our stomach capacity is also customized to our unique physical frame by using our own hand measurements too. Four hand measurements per meal is a good estimation. Therefore, in the guide below, "your" refers to whoever is doing the eating.

Most veggies, fruits, and grains can be measured by using your **fist** or **open hand** as a guide:

- One serving of veggies or fruit is about the size of your fist.

- One serving of cereal, pasta, or brown rice is about the size of your fist.

- One serving of bagels or muffins is about the size of your fist.

- One serving of raw leafy greens is about the size of your two cupped hands.

- One serving of bread is about the thickness and size of your open hand, up to the first row of knuckles above your ring finger.

Most protein foods can be measured by using the **palm** as a guide:

- One serving of meat is about the size of your entire palm including its thickness.

- One serving of beans, peas, or lentils is about the size of your entire palm including its thickness.

- One serving of shelled nuts, seeds or peanut butter is about the size of the *surface* of your palm.

Most dairy products can be measured by using **three parts** of the hand as a guide:

- One serving of milk or yogurt is about the size of your fist.

- One serving of sliced cheese is about the size of the surface of your palm.

- One serving of block cheese is about the size of your entire thumb.

The next question is how many hand portions per day? The *average* adult's stomach capacity can hold about four cups (one quart) of food and drink. In the Old Testament, the Hebrew people were instructed to gather approximately eight cups (two quarts) of manna per person, to eat throughout the day. Even with all the walking they did, this amount kept them alive and thriving throughout their forty year journey.

Most people today would find this amount too small, so even if we upped the number to twelve cups (three quarts) of ***quality*** food per day, most people would still be eating fewer calories than they are right now, as long as they were eating whole, real food.

Over three-fourths of the food on your plate should come from a plant: Veggies, fruits, beans, peas, lentils, and whole grains. The government website, choosemyplate.gov, advises that you fill half of your plate with lots of veggies and fruits. Just over one-fourth of the remaining plate should be filled with whole grains such as bread, rice, or pasta. The remaining (slightly less than) one-fourth of the plate should be lean protein. All people, nine-years-old and over, should have three cups of milk or the equivalent in dairy products each day.

Obviously, there will be some fluctuation in this routine. If you eat a meal with extra brown rice, there will be more grain on the plate and less of something else, such as fruit. If you don't eat fruit with every meal, you might eat that serving later on for a snack. Learn to balance things out by moving them to another meal or snack. When in doubt always assume that you need more vegetables or fruits, because most people don't eat enough of them.

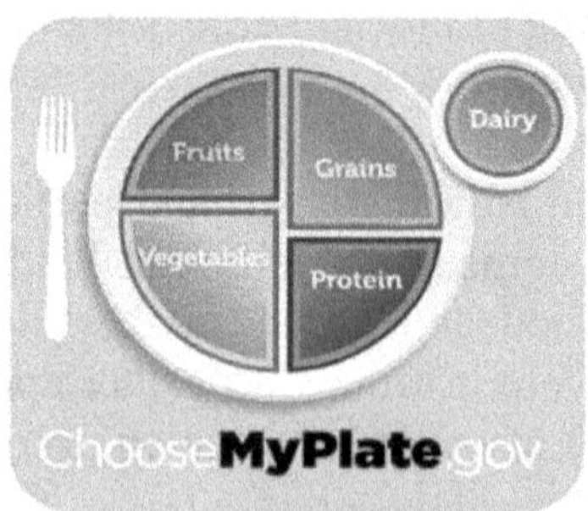

If you use this model for your structured mealtimes, three times a day, every day, it will help ensure that your children are receiving adequate nutrients. They will also be closer to reaping the following benefits within a short amount of time.

- ✓ They will lose weight if they are overweight.
- ✓ They will be taking powerful steps toward living a healthy life.
- ✓ They will be closer to reaching their daily nutritional requirements.
- ✓ They will be closer to eating and drinking within their calorie range.
- ✓ They will be taking powerful steps toward extending their longevity.
- ✓ They will be improving the level of their self-image, because the healthier and leaner your children become, the more their confidence will grow.
- ✓ They will be improving the quality of their lives, not only physically, but also mentally, emotionally and socially. Because the clearer they think and the better they feel, the more they'll learn and the happier they'll be, all of which has the potential to improve their social lives.

All of these suggestions are merely guidelines. They are by no means perfect measurements, but they are good estimations based on reliable sources. By using the hand to measure your food portions, you will be closer to eating the correct serving sizes, rather than taking a shot in the dark.

The bottom line is that an active child can eat almost anything, in any amount in the nutritious food groups, as long as it's not covered in cream, sizzled in grease, smothered in butter or soaked in sugar, because energetic kids burn off calories quickly. It's the unhealthy additions and preparation that can turn a good food into a bad food.

Serve food on a smaller plate for younger children. An easy way to remember these portion sizes is to use plates with dividers for your children. For more information on serving sizes, visit choosemyplate.gov/food-groups.

STRATEGY 4: THE ACTIVE INTERACTIVE PLAN

This takes us to the fourth point of why the ways of antiquity worked in maintaining ideal weight. People were more physically active and more socially interactive on a *face-to-face basis*. They found meaningful things to do with their lives that were interesting, fulfilling, and fun. This meant that they were rarely bored, even in times of quiet.

Losing weight and gaining health and quality of life is all about changing behaviors. The second half of this book is designed to do just that with hundreds of ideas and suggestions. Overcoming an opponent can often be done by simply turning around, walking away, and finding something else to do.

I'M BORED!

DIRECT YOUR THOUGHTS AND ACTIONS

Feeding the mind healthy and uplifting "food" nourishes the soul and empowers a person to walk a higher path. The activities listed in the second half of this book are intended to create new ideas and diversions that will block, distract, or drive out thoughts that lead to unhealthy eating and unproductive living. When the hands and feet are busily involved in interesting activities, they're not busy feeding the mouth or chasing after meaningless pursuits.

This isn't to say that a child should be in a perpetual state of motion. On the contrary, children need time to rest and relax every day. But even in their downtimes, they can engage their minds in productive pleasures such as reading, writing, journaling, and drawing, playing an instrument, or listening to spiritual, classical, or other types of soothing music. These quieter activities help rejuvenate their bodies, focus their minds, and sustain their spirits.

TRUE HUNGER VERSUS BOREDOM

It's no secret that people eat when they are bored. Perceived hunger and tedium often go hand-in-hand, or rather hand-to-mouth. Many parents will often tell a bored child to go outside and play or find something constructive to do. The problem is that many children don't know what to do, so they take the path of least resistance and revert to their usual routine: Flop in front of the TV, connect on the internet, or play video games, often while snacking on candy or junk food during these sedentary activities. In extreme cases of boredom, or lack of direction in the fun department, many kids look for excitement in negative ways by drinking alcohol, taking drugs, causing mischief, or getting into trouble.

Children need to see that there's a great big world outside their media screens, if they'll only unplug and step out of their virtual world and into the real world to experience it. Life outside of cyberspace is a great place to explore the world in real time with real people. When children have more face-to-face interactions there are fewer hand-to-mouth interactions, as long as the meetings don't involve eating unhealthy food. As parents and caregivers, we can help children discover what their interests are and then point them in the right direction to help them develop their natural skills, talents, and abilities that nurture their emotions, bodies, and brains.

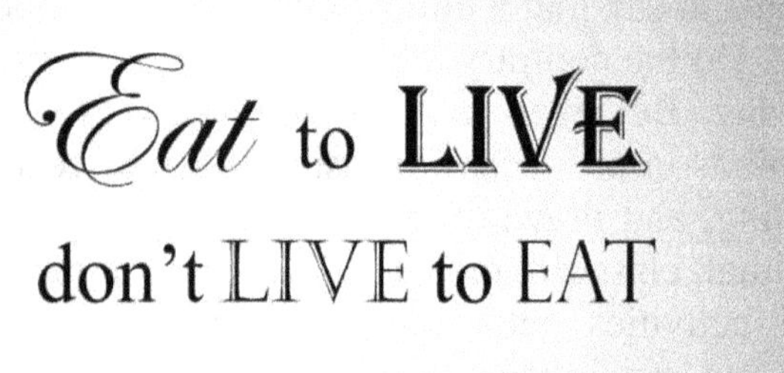

When children are busy living interesting lives, and when they view food as nourishment to sustain life, rather than an epicenter of entertainment, they will not be a slave to its rule. When life is full of new and enjoyable adventures, and the mind is engaged in thoughtful endeavors, junk food loses its power to control a person's behavior.

This is because the brain is the source of all thoughts and ideas that lead to deeds. No matter how well you multi-task, you can only think one thought at a time. Therefore, just as two objects cannot occupy the same space, positive thoughts that lead to virtuous habits cannot coexist with negative thoughts that lead to hazardous habits. In the same way, obsessive thoughts *about* food usually lead to compulsive actions *to eat* food, since thoughts always precede deeds.

It's true that losing weight is a numbers game that we can win. It's also true that productivity brings its own reward, but there must be a lifestyle change to attain these crowns. To get the tiara atop your head, you must begin *inside* your head. What you fill your noggin with, by way of what you see and hear, is what will manifest in your life through your words and actions. The old computer programming slogan that says, "Garbage in, garbage out," pertains to the mind too. Everything that enters your brain influences how you act. To change a behavior, you must change your thoughts. The way to change your thoughts is by using caution and care when choosing what goes into your brain via your eyes and ears.

MISBEHAVIOR IS OFTEN DUE TO BOREDOM

Children often misbehave or whine when they want more of your time and attention, or when they are tired, hungry, or bored. It's easy to make a quick evaluation to discover the source of their frustration: If a child is well-fed, well-rested, and well-nurtured then he's probably bored and doesn't know how to occupy himself. A child isn't deliberately acting up to tick you off. Well, maybe sometimes. Most of the time, he or she is doing it because kids of all ages and all walks of life need stimulation to feed their growing minds.

When there's no one to connect to, or no goal to shoot for, or when their aim is headed in the wrong direction or down a negative path (and then halted by your roadblocks), children often spin in circles of anger, frustration, or defiance.

This innate desire to connect, or to hone in on a target is why texting, social sites, and electronic games and gadgets are so addictive. Children feed this emotional or goal-seeking need via online screens, because there's always a message to send, a score to beat, or a virtual prize to attain. The device often poses a challenge that provides immediate feedback and a bit of temporal pleasure. This behavior alone indicates that children are not only up for physical challenges, but also those with emotional and mental incentives too.

With a little effort you can nudge them in the right direction, not only with playtime, but also with projects or even a bit of work. Most children, when engaged in something productive that truly interests them, are happy and well-behaved. The key is finding and pressing the right buttons that light up their lives and rev their engines.

A good rule to establish for your children is no electronic entertainment or television until they've done something to strengthen their bodies or develop their brains. Sedentary amusement should be "dessert" after the main course of physical activity, creative play, or challenges that stimulate the mind. The way to adhere to this rule is to control the portal to cyberspace. Set limits on TV, PC, and cell phone use, and any other doorways to the virtual world. Withhold electronic entertainment until they have walked, biked, read, created, or done some other type of constructive activity for *at least* one hour a day. Since you pay the electric bill (and probably the cell phone bill), you have a right to control the on/off switch to these devices. They may think that you're being mean, but you are really redirecting their focus for their own good, so they can better their lives and learn amazing things.

Many of the activities suggested in this book are free or fairly affordable. The ones that cost a little bit more can be managed by taking the money spent on junk food and frivolous fluff and using it for day trips to museums, gorges, falls, and other places of interest. Don't bother with big ticket toys that light up and make noise, or the electronics that offer no real satisfaction or education. Buy your children a telescope, take them to a play, or buy inspiring books to read that spark their imaginations. Take them places that will fill their minds with creative ideas. The zoo is fine. Camping is great, but how about a museum or a skills workshop? Most children will have an awesome time and learn something new in the process.

HOW TO REIN IN OVEREATING

Most overweight and obese children suffer emotionally due to rejection, depression, bullying, and feelings of inferiority. This section is for them, and for those of you who have ever struggled to the point of tears, and for those who have ever tried everything there is to lose weight, only to fail again-and-again in the process. What I am about to say is a doable way to help you or your child break this vicious cycle, so when the scales tip in your favor, you gain *better health, a leaner physique, and a happier life* in its place.

I used these methods myself, along with the first three strategies, *eat nutritious food, eat at scheduled times, eat appropriate portions sizes*, to overcome my own eating dysfunctions and weight issues. What I am about to share will teach you how to stick to scheduled mealtimes, and at the same time, incorporate the fourth strategy of becoming more physically active and more socially interactive.

On the following pages you will find hundreds of ideas listing all types of things to do. As you read the remainder of this book, write down any and all suggestions that interest you *that can be done on a moment's notice,* or any project that you can begin and then *return to, on a moment's notice.* The list should consist of at least twenty-five *or more* fun, educational, or productive activities, such as taking a walk, painting your fingernails, arranging tools, watering plants, organizing drawers, washing the car, or returning to an ongoing project. Add any sports or games to play, if someone is around to do them with you. Jot down things such as drawing, sewing, writing, or doing a good deed for someone.

This is one of the greatest secrets that reined in my out-of-control eating habits and helped me win the victory. Are you ready? Here it is: Once you have written down your personal list of things to do, keep it with you *at all times.* Put it in your pocket, tuck it in your wallet, or stuff it in your shoe, just don't go anywhere without this list even when you are home. Keep it with you *at all times if you want to improve your life and get a handle on your eating habits*! Rewrite it when it's ripped, iron it when it's wrinkled, frame it if you must, but keep this list nearby because *it is your escape hatch* to keep you from boredom, stress, and emotional eating. You cannot fight your temptations and win without some type of strategy. You cannot control your temptations and win without a plan of action. *You must get away from your temptations by replacing them with something else in order to be victorious.*

The bottom line is that unless it is breakfast, lunch, dinner, or a light evening snack, you should not be eating food or sipping calorie-laden drinks. Instead of the usual in-between meal picking, you're going to pick up your list instead. Check it twice if you must, but then *immediately* pray and get away from the source of temptation, and get busy doing the activity you have chosen from your list until the desire passes. If the desire doesn't pass with one activity, choose another one, and follow through. Do this until the behavior becomes second nature and you will eventually get a handle on this issue and lose weight. But you must stick to the entire program: *eat nutritious food, eat at scheduled times, eat appropriate portions sizes, and use your list in-between to become more physically, mentally, and socially active.*

This also means don't eat food while cooking it. When you are ready to eat a meal, put your portions in front of you before you begin to eat, then when you are done, you are done. Get up and do something else, but don't eat leftovers when you put them away. You are not a waste-basket.

Continue to revise and update the list as you cross off activities once they're completed. These diversions create new habits, which build inner-strength and bring inner-satisfaction and confidence. Not only that, but you will also be doing something productive in the process. Positive activities keep food from becoming an escape or the main source of pleasure and entertainment, since most eating between meals is often boredom disguised as hunger. This method works because repeatedly doing positive deeds has a way of pushing out negative habits.

NOTE: Think of yourself as an athlete in training. You may not "get it" the first time, but keep at it. You wouldn't expect to master a sport the very first time you tried, and this is no exception. It's normal to fall but expect success, so pick yourself up, dust yourself off, and get back in the game.

DISCOVER YOUR INNER CHILD

Someone once said that we don't stop playing because we grow old. We grow old because we stop playing. Dr. Stuart Brown said, "Those who play rarely become brittle in the face of stress or lose the healing capacity for humor." Jesus taught that we must become like little children to enter the kingdom of heaven. A foretaste of bliss right here on earth is possible, if we humble ourselves like these wee little ones.

Children don't worry about looking silly when they are having fun. They're not concerned about things that bog adults down like collecting more stuff to impress other people, or putting on airs to appear more important. If not for commercials and comparisons (of their playthings to other kids' toys), children would be completely content with simple pleasures and nature's treasures. They'd find things to do with sticks and stones and puddles of mud. They'd stop mid-stride to stare at clouds, pick up bugs, or twirl in circles of joy, and then giggle themselves to sleep at night. Another day merely means another adventure for them.

Little children also possess pure faith. They don't think about the past or worry about the future. They live in the present moment. Someone once said that you'll find more happiness growing down than up. Granted, we need adults to make contributions to society for its benefit, but we also need to take time to unwind. A bow must be unstrung on occasion or the string will lose its elasticity and usefulness. In the same way, childlike playfulness adds a spring to our step, a joy to our status quo, and a brightness to our future.

Children give us an excuse to act silly and play, but this simplicity requires humility and vulnerability. It may not be an easy trait to attain, but it's worth every ounce of the effort. A strong bond of love is formed when adults play with their children, not only games and sports, but also in everyday interactions.

LITTLE TYKES

Keeping healthy and fit should be so fun and enjoyable that it becomes part of your child's daily routine. Children ages 2-5 merely need to play to stay in shape. There's really no set amount of time that they should spend being active, because kids at this age are always on the go. It's usually more of a chore to get them to sit still.

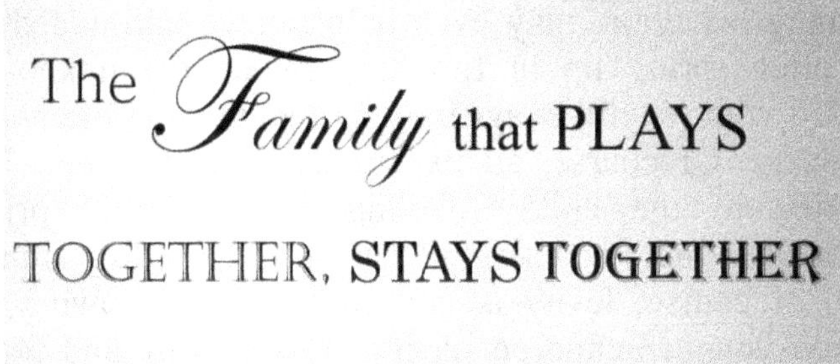

Everything seems to pique a child's curiosity and grab his or her attention at this age. The challenge as they grow is to find positive outlets to keep their minds and bodies busy. Of course, there's always the playground where they can swing and slide and crawl through those hamster-like tubes, or the traditional games of hide-and-seek, or tag, or a trip to the kiddie pool. If you don't have a swimming pool, sprinkler, or hose in your yard, fill the bathtub with water and let young children hop in wearing their swimsuits. Toss in a few toys and let them play in the "pool" on hot days. Obviously, they should be well supervised, always within your line of vision, just as they would be if outside in a real pool.

Another way to keep tots occupied is to fill a large wide-based plastic bowl or dish tub halfway up with water, place it on a bath towel on a table or the floor, and use it as a swimming pool for small plastic dolls, or an ocean for little fish or boats. Add a few accessories to their pool party and they will play for hours.

MAKE IT FUN AND LEARNING WILL COME

Some of the following silly antics are things I've done with my own children. I'm still a kid at heart when it comes to having fun and making children smile and laugh. I love to tease and exaggerate, or make it seem like they got something over on me, which may also build their self-esteem. Humor is also a great shock absorber to help them over the bumps in life. Some of these goofy games and clowning behaviors may even help relieve unfounded fears that often spring up in tiny tots. When the unknown is handled with playful exaggeration, the situation often seems less scary. Of course, all experiences are different. Being sensitive to the child's feelings is always a priority, especially if there is a serious fear or an unsettling situation. Then, of course, levity is not fitting. The following ideas provide younger children plenty of your time and focused attention to make them feel cherished and special.

1. Playtime with plastic food can be both fun and educational. Sort the food items into groups and then get into character of the maître d' or the customer. For dining out, make a simple menu from a folded sheet of paper and then act out the scene as the head waiter or waitress. Ham it up as you say, "Good evening, madam (or sir). Welcome to Fido's

Restaurant (use a silly name such as their pet's or a favorite toy). Please follow me to your table." Add an exaggerated walk, pull out a chair, and say, "You may be seated here," and then hand each child a menu, write down the order, and then off you go. The sillier the experience the better. When you serve them, "accidently" drop the plastic food on them, and apologize profusely while pretending to wipe the spill with a napkin. While "buttering" a slice of plastic bread, act as though distracted while talking to them, and then "butter" your hand or both sides of the bread. Appear to be thoroughly flustered when you realize your mistake. This usually produces a gaggle of giggles.

The educational part of the food play can be done by taking the serious route and learning good table manners. I prefer the silly route though, since we are indeed playing with very small children. It also lessens feelings of self-consciousness if they should make an error in etiquette while eating a real meal. When you are finished playing, you can teach them about nutrition when you put the food away. As each item goes back into the box, ask the child if that particular food helps them grow healthy and strong, or if it does not.

Another version of this restaurant playtime can be done while preparing real lunch for your children. Spread a tablecloth on the living room floor and have an indoor picnic. Make a "menu" on a plain sheet of paper listing healthy lunch or snack choices, and then categorize them like a real carte du jour.

- Main course: Peanut butter and honey sandwich, turkey and veggies on whole grain bread, scrambled eggs with whole grain toast, mini-pizza on whole grain pocket bread.
- Veggies: baby carrots, cherry tomatoes, cucumbers, green beans.

- Fruit: bananas, strawberries, apple slices, melon, berries.
- Beverages: milk, juice, fruit smoothie, water.
- Dessert: 100% frozen juice pop, whole grain Fig Newton cookie, read a story, play a game.

You get the idea. Add whatever healthy foods you have on hand. Pretend you are the waitress and serve them lunch with much flair and fanfare. Use your best accent and then carry their order to them on a tray. Another version is to serve lunch or dinner on fancy dishes and then eat by candlelight. Put a vase of flowers on the table to enhance their dining experience. This will also teach them the importance of loving service and setting an attractive table.

2. Play hide-and-seek with a silly slant. This works well with a small child who doesn't quite know how to hide well yet. Here's the set-up. The child (usually 2 through 4 years old) hides somewhere where you can obviously see him and he can easily see you. The goofy part of this game is that you look in ridiculous places for him such as in a drawer, a cupboard, or a plant, all the while calling out the child's name: "Where could Joey be? Is he in the plant?" (Peek into the leafy plant) "Noooo, not there." Act frustrated as you move to the drawer, "Maybe he's in the drawer!" (Open a small drawer and look inside. Rummage through a few things, and you should hear the child laughing.) Stop and muse, "Hummmm, I know! He's in the cupboard!" (Hurry to the cupboard like you've finally figured it out, and then fling the door wide open). "NOPE! He's not in there!" Stomp your foot in mock frustration. By now, the child should be laughing hysterically. Proclaim that you can hear him, but then walk in the opposite direction, and say, "I know! He's in my shoe!" Pick up the shoe, turn it over and shake it, demanding that the child come out. When the laughing gets even more hysterical, "find" the child. This game may end up

being more fun for you than for the child when you hear the shrieks of laughter.

Another way to make this game silly for a younger child (who knows how to count to ten) is when it is your turn to count, and their turn to hide, pretend that you forgot how to recite the numbers in order. Call them off in random order, very slow and loud: "1, 2, 5, 8, 4, 7…" This also produces snickers and giggles. When you find the child, have him teach you how to count properly and act enlightened when he tells you.

3. When the child introduces you to a new stuffed animal, act as though you're having a hard time remembering its name. An elephant named Peanut then becomes, "Pickles? Petunia? Oh! Wait! I remember! It's Walnut!"

4. When a child sits down to eat a bowl of soup or cereal, hand him a very large serving spoon. When he looks puzzled or laughs, act surprised that you gave him the spoon, as though you had no idea where it came from, or how it got in your hand. Apologize profusely and then give him a regular spoon.

5. Draw a smiley face on a grapefruit with a black Sharpie marker and give it to a child when he or she is sick in bed. Set it where they can easily see it while they're recuperating.

6. When a young child is in the bathtub, give him a mound of shaving cream to lather on his cheeks and chin, and then let him "shave" it off with a teaspoon.

7. Hide a small plastic toy (about 2 inches tall) and have the child look for it. Inform the child when he's cold, warm, hot, or boiling, as he gets closer or further from the hidden object. Have them ask for clues, such as *is it high like a bird or low like a snake?*

8. Gather up about ten small toys and place them in a pile then have the child study them. After a moment have the child leave the room, as you hide one of the items behind your back. When the child returns, ask him or her which item is missing.

9. Have two or three children sit on the bottom step of a staircase. Place a coin in one hand and close both hands into a fist. Show both fists to each child and let each one choose a hand to find the coin. If the child is correct, he or she moves up one step. Do this for each child until one of them reaches the top.

10. Hide a small toy and then draw a treasure map with paces for them to follow until they reach the "X" that marks the spot where the "treasure" is hidden. Modify the hunt when playing outside.

11. Cover a cardboard paper towel roll with foil to create a makeshift microphone and host a pretend interview. Ask young children basic questions such as their name, favorite color, what they like to do, and what their favorite toy is. When it's the child's turn to ask you questions, give them silly or ridiculous answers, make up an alien language, or speak in a foreign accent to make the interview as silly as possible.

12. Teach young children how to identify the letters of the alphabet by calling them out in random order as they type each letter on a keyboard. Have them type words into a search engine and then click on images to view photos of nature, animals, and sea life online.

13. Have young children point to items in the room or in a picture book that begin with each letter of the alphabet.

14. Pick up a few large cardboard boxes from an appliance store and build a little village in your own backyard. Have the children cut out windows and doors to make a house, cottage, castle, or fort. Paint stones or brick designs on each building. Or open the boxes up and cut out holes for faces, and then paint silly bodies under each hole, such as clowns, cowboys, or southern bells with parasols. Be sure to take lots of pictures.

15. Rotate your children's toys to make them seem new again. Box up a group of toys or games and put them away for a few months. When you bring them out again to play, put another group of them away.

16. Plug your children into free online learning games such as pbskids.org and starfall.com. Find fun printout activities at theyarelearning.com. An affordable fun app for preschoolers that teaches life skills is the *Dr. Panda* series. Each game takes a child through processes that pertain to daily living or potential careers such as running a home, restaurant, airport, garage, daycare, hospital, veggie garden, handyman service, supermarket, preschool learning, classroom, art class, or beauty salon.

17. Surround your children with art supplies and learning toys such as Legos, building blocks, clay, and Play-Doh. Give them an assortment of tools to work with such as rolling pins, cookie cutters, plastic cutlery and spatulas. Recipes abound online for homemade play dough, flubber and other goopy-glop type concoctions that can be molded and shaped for hours. Involve kids in preparing the mixtures as well as playing with the end results.

WHISTLE WHILE YOU WORK

Giving children fun learning experiences and a measure of responsibility will enrich their minds and develop their lives for future independence and service to others. The following suggestions, not only give the child an education, but also a feeling of purpose and meaning. It is important to work alongside your children on a regular basis, since you are their greatest role model at this point in their lives.

> In bringing up CHILDREN,
> spend on them HALF as much money and
> twice as much time
>
> UNKNOWN

Brian Sutton-Smith, a play theorist of the late 20th century, said that the opposite of play is not work. It's depression. Work is often playtime to a child. We see this when they imitate adults. If you look at their make-believe activities, many of them are spent mimicking jobs that grown-ups do. We see this when they play house, pretend to cook, sweep the floor, or care for a baby doll; or when they become detectives to spy on bad guys, or mechanics to repair cars that look a lot like bikes. Mary Poppins famously said, "In every job that must be done, there is an element of fun." Work can be fun, enjoyable, or fulfilling. It all depends on a person's attitude, which can be shaped at an early age with positive feedback and praise.

Make jobs such as picking up toys or pulling weeds a fun competition, a race, or a challenge for boys and girls. Set a timer to see who finishes first or who gets the most done. We see this measure of competition as a motivating force in the workplace via commission, piecework, or high numbers on paychecks. Friendly competition motivates people to perform better, yet the sole aim beneath this one-upping should be that of having fun and practicing good sportsmanship.

Use checklists for chores or star charts for completed projects to keep children motivated, and to help them keep track of their progress. Check marks, stars, and stickers are forms of visual praise. When you acknowledge their progress and praise your children for doing a good job or for being good helpers, they will be encouraged to work more willingly and diligently in the future.

Most young children enjoy working alongside an adult. It may be work to you, but it is companionship and fun camaraderie to them. When you make work enjoyable, they will associate it with love and happy memories. The following are ways a child can help out.

- Help rinse dishes.

- Water plants or the garden.

- Sweep the sidewalk or floor.

- Dust, make a bed, fold clothes, or rake leaves.

- Place library books on the desk to check them out.

- Add ingredients to a bowl when cooking or baking.

- Sort and organize silverware into the correct compartments when putting away clean dishes. They can also sort and organize pots and pans, plastic bowls, and canned goods in the cupboards.

- Hand the gas station attendant the cash when he pumps the fuel. This helps a child associate money with products and services, and see that fuel is not magically downloaded into the tank. Let them do the same with cashiers in the store.

- Hold the cap and pour laundry soap into the washer. Let them help transfer the clothes from the washer to the dryer. To make this fun, "miss" their hands and put a washcloth on their arm or head instead, and then teasingly say, "Oooops! I am so sorry!" This usually produces laughter and giggles, and they'll often want to help even more.

Make a game of small jobs and have fun while doing them. Sing or whistle a happy tune. Make up or sing silly songs while you work. Ask them what the next step is in the process of cooking, cleaning, or laundry. Act as though they are teaching you. Pretend to get it wrong and let them show you how to do it right, and then praise them for being so smart. Create a lot of fanfare when they enlighten you. Say something like, "Ohhhhh, now I see! Thank you for showing me!" or "You are so smart! Good job!" When you give a child age-appropriate work to do, it will raise their self-esteem.

DESIGN YOUR ADVENTURES

At one time, kids spent hours outside playing with things like bats and balls or looking for critters like bugs and toads. They skated, hiked, and biked until the streetlights came on at night. And because of these passionate activities, children were rarely bored or overweight.

Not so much today. The effects of a sedentary lifestyle are obvious to see wherever we happen to look. Children need mental stimulation and creative play, and at least one hour of energetic physical activity every day for healthy brain, heart, and lung function and to maintain an ideal weight.

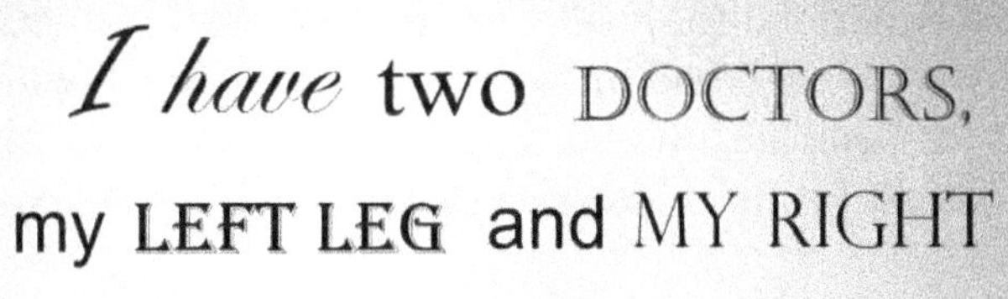

Children can easily build and strengthen their bones and muscles by doing simple things like running, jumping, pushing, pulling, climbing, and crawling around any recreational area. If you envisioned a playground as a mini-fitness center, you'd happily pay to get them in shape, but it's absolutely free to take them there and do the aforementioned activities.

Regular physical activity generates new growth and development of nerve tissue in the brain. A proper diet and exercise also controls blood-sugar levels and helps insulin work more efficiently in the body by delivering glucose to the cells. Aside from the obvious toning, strengthening, and weight loss attributed to exercise, a vigorous workout or playtime reduces anxiety, boosts immunity, improves sleep, and enhances memory and brain function.

Strenuous exercise floods the brain with the feel good hormone dopamine. It also releases those lovely mood-enhancing endorphins that reduce pain and increase feelings of well-being. If you keep kids hopping to get those hormones popping, there will come a time when they will feel uncomfortable *not* running, jumping, or skipping in some way, shape, or form. When kids enjoy what they're doing, they will "play" longer with greater enthusiasm and intensity, and look forward to doing the activities again.

Walking

Two of the most basic forms of transportation are also two of the most beneficial for health and fitness. Walking and biking both involve vigorous movement of the legs, which are crucial for heart health and lung function. They are also two of the easiest forms of exercise to incorporate into your life.

My parents owned one car when I was growing up, so my sister and I walked almost everywhere we needed to go, no matter what the temperature or weather (aside from an occasional ride during sub-zero temps and torrential rains). We weren't chauffeured around town to attend events or to meet with our friends and most of our friends weren't chauffeured either. "Mom and Pop" taxi services weren't around in the 60s and 70s.

As a result, we trudged to school, to the store, to visit relatives, or to meet friends dressed for the weather as we ventured out. While we walked, we caught snowflakes on our tongues and threw snowballs in the winter. We picked wildflowers in fields and splashed through puddles in the spring. We raced our bikes down dirt paths and ran through lawn sprinklers in the summer. We rustled our feet through piles of leaves and collected horse-chestnuts in the fall. We saw sights we never would have seen, if we had been driven to our destinations.

The one-to-eight miles I walked almost daily from third grade through high school, kept me in shape, deepened my relationships, made me aware of my surroundings, and gave me an appreciation of nature. Walking gave me time to chat with my sister or friends, while breathing the crisp morning air or the cool evening breeze, all of which were invigorating and made me feel alive. Walking by myself gave me time to ponder things going on in my life. It cleared the cobwebs from my head and gave me clarity of thought.

Walking was fun and refreshing, and I felt great while doing it, but I didn't realize its benefits until many years and pounds later, after I had given it up in exchange for driving a car. I eventually noticed and missed the physical, mental, and emotional perks that walking and biking had bestowed upon me during my younger years, so I eventually took them up again.

To gain the most health benefits, walk as many places as you can to get where you need to go. Choose functional and comfortable over fashionable when buying a pair of walking or jogging shoes. Walking should be done at a steady pace. A slow saunter is better than nothing, but if you want to lose weight, strengthen your heart and lungs, and reap the mental and emotional benefits, you must walk at a fairly good clip. The speed should be the intensity of someone who is hurrying to catch a bus or trying to get to class on time. You've passed the pace test if you can hustle your butt and hold a conversation at the same time without sounding winded.

Be sure the areas where you walk are safe, well-lit, and out in the open, ideally with other people nearby. Do not walk in the wee hours of the morning or in the darkness of night when no one is around to help you, should you have an emergency. If you must walk in the road, walk *facing* traffic. Walkers always travel in the opposite direction of wheels. For more tips on walking safely visit www.walkinginfo.org.

Biking

All of the health benefits that apply to walking also apply to biking. Children should learn to ride a tricycle as soon as they are able to push the pedals. A child should be over ten years-old before he rides a bike in the road. Bikers should always ride with the flow of traffic and obey the same rules of the road as cars, trucks, and motorcycles. An easy way to remember which direction to ride a bike in the road is that all wheels travel in the same direction.

The National Highway Traffic Safety Administration advises that bikers wear a properly fitted helmet. They should also wear neon, fluorescent, or other bright colors (not white) when riding day or night. If older children ride at night, they should wear something that reflects light or they should have flashing lights on their bicycles.

Encourage your children to bike wherever they need to go for the same reasons previously listed for walking. More bicycle safety tips can be found at www.nhtsa.gov/bicycles.

Calling

When out and about in public places, there are few things more terrifying than losing a child in a crowd (or anywhere else for that matter). If you're going to be amid the masses with small children, there are a few things you can do to keep track of them. Dress your children in similar or bright colored shirts, so they are easy to spot in a crowd. Write your name and cell phone number (with the area code) on a small piece of paper and tuck it into each child's pocket. Tell the child that if he or she should become separated from you, to hand the number to someone in charge, such as a uniformed policeman, a security guard, or a clerk wearing a nametag. That way, the person can call to let you know where your child is so you can pick him or her up.

Teach children their full names, your name, and your phone number. Another tip is to take a picture of each child with your cell phone before you go out. If a child should become lost, you'll have a photo of him or her to use as an identifier, to show people and police what the child looks like and what he or she is wearing so they can help find the child. The photo can also be shared quickly with other police to help locate the child.

Once a child can recognize numbers and understand the concept, teach them how to call 911 in case of an emergency.

ACTIVITIES OF CHASE, RACE, AND PACE

Old-fashioned outdoor games are usually free to play and easy to learn. Teach your children some of the games that you used to play when you were young. Encourage them to join a sports team, an organization, or a club. The commitment and camaraderie will teach them responsibility, dedication, and perseverance.

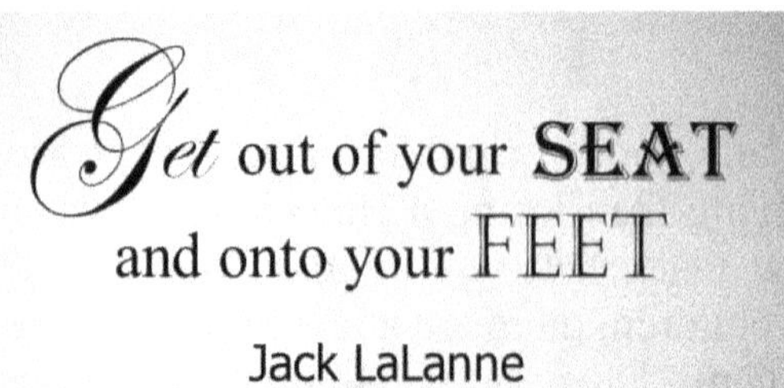

I've listed the following games that I used to play and enjoy as a child, along with quite a few others. If you don't know how to play these games, you can find detailed instructions on the web. Tap into your inner child and join in the fun.

Classic Acts

Duck, Duck, Goose!
Hide-and-Seek
Hopscotch
Kick the Can
Mother, May I?
Musical Chairs
Red Light, Green Light
Red Rover
Simon Says
Spud!
Tag / Freeze Tag / TV Tag

Spinnin' your Wheels!

Biking
Hula hoop
Roller-skating
Skateboarding

Slidin' and Glidin'!

Cross-country Skiing
Ice hockey

Ice skating
Skateboarding
Sledding / tobogganing
Snow Skiing
Snow tubing
Snowboarding

Leapin' Lizards!

Jump rope / Double Dutch
Obstacle course (make your own)
Rebounder (mini-trampoline)
Stepper
Trampoline (enclosed with net)

Hit it!

Air hockey
Badminton
Baseball
Billiards
Bocce Ball
Bowling
Boxing
Cricket
Croquet
Foosball
Golf / miniature golf
Hacky Sack
Lacrosse
Ping pong
Racquetball
Softball
Street hockey
T-ball
Tennis
Volleyball
Wiffle ball

Catch Me if You Can!

Basketball
Dodge ball
Football / Touch football
Frisbee
Kickball
Ring Toss
Rugby
Soccer
Track / Hurdles
Wrestling

Splish Splash!

Boating
Fishing
Slip 'n' Slide
Surfing
Swimming
Wading in a creek
Water-skiing
Wind-surfing

Shake A Leg!

Ballet
Cheerleading
Gymnastics
Pilates
Tap Dancing
Yoga
Zumba

More Boredom Busters!

Build a snowman
Build an igloo, snow fort, or snow cave

Collect beach glass
Collect coins
Collect rocks and minerals
Fly a glider
Fly a kite
Go horseback riding
Go rock climbing
Go to a circus
Go to a county fair
Go to a dog show
Go to a rodeo
Lift weights
Play Wii Fitness games like boxing and jogging
Roll coins and be on the lookout for old ones
Skip rocks on a pond or lake
Visit a pet shop

Encourage kids to play outside, not only in the warm sunshine, but also in the snow, wind, and rain. Bundle them up in the winter and show them how to make snow angels. Slip on a pair of boots, grab an umbrella, and then walk, splash, or dance with them in the rain.

CRAFTY KIDS

Encourage your children make birthday or Christmas gifts for friends and family members. These presents are often the gifts that are cherished and treasured by teachers, grandparents, and aunts and uncles.

Most of the supplies needed below can be found in the craft section of department stores. Some of them are prepackaged as kits. Many of these ideas and many more projects can be found on YouTube tutorials. You can also find loads of crafty and artistic ideas on Pinterest.

- Build a fort
- Finger paint
- Paint T-shirts
- Make jewelry
- Arrange flowers
- Make a rain stick
- Build a birdhouse
- Learn to do origami
- Do rubber stamp art
- Make a messenger bag
- Paint a mural on a wall
- Make latch-hook pillows
- Make potholders with loops
- Make rainbow loom jewelry
- Tie-dye scarves, clothes, or curtains
- Make snowflakes from folded white paper
- Make a ribbon crown or a daisy chain crown
- Make a set of wind chimes with old keys, bottles, or silverware

- Make jewelry from old skeleton keys, small washers, or vintage buttons

- Make clay imprints of hands, leaves, or flowers and then paint them

- Paint designs on your fingernails such as bumblebees, ladybugs, or flowers

- Paint premade wooden toys, letters, or birdhouses found in a store's craft section

- Make a necklace holder from pretty or old dresser knobs attached to a small board

- Attend a craft show, or create something and then become a vendor at a craft show

- Paint animals, insects, flowers, names, quotes, or other designs onto stones or slate

- Spray paint small stones gold to make "gold nuggets." Hide them in the yard and then host a treasure hunt. Sew small pouches for each child to collect and store his or her gold

ACTIVITIES, ORGANIZATIONS, AND CLUBS

Activities, organizations and clubs can give a child of sense of belonging. The experience may also teach a child how to work with a group of people toward a common goal. Some of these groups require teamwork and unity to accomplish their purposes. These are qualities that children can draw upon in the future when entering the workplace or training for careers.

- Join a marching band
- Join a pottery or a ceramics class
- Join your local YMCA or YWCA
- Try out for a school play or musical
- Join a church or church youth group
- Join a Bible study or prayer meeting
- Join a debate team or a public speaking group
- Join your local Boys & Girls Club of America ww.bgca.org
- Join a photography club and then enter your photos in contests
- Join the 4-H Youth Development Program. Find out more at 4-h.org
- Run for student council, class secretary, treasurer, vice president, or president
- Join Future Farmers of American at www.ffa.org. "FFA makes a positive difference in the lives of students by developing their potential for premier leadership, personal growth, and career success through agricultural education."

MAKE ONE DAY A WEEK FUNDAY

Make one day a week specifically a "Funday" to relax or do something special with family or friends. Make it simple or elaborate by planning a mini-daycation at home, in the yard, or somewhere nearby. You can also find more things to do by going to www.boredomMD.com and search for events in your area.

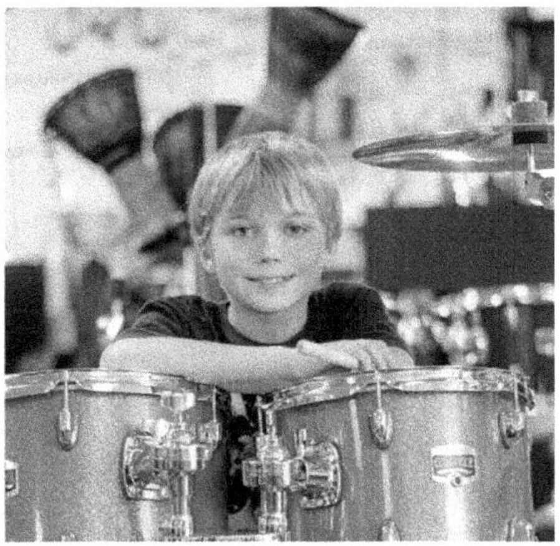

Go!

- Attend a parade
- Visit a petting zoo
- Attend an antique car show
- Attend a historical reenactment
- Rent a go cart then go for a ride
- See a Festival of Lights show at Christmastime
- Attend cooking classes and events at groceries stores such as Wegmans
- Attend fairs, festivals, parks, carnivals, and other city or county celebrations

- Attend a free kid's class at Michael's Arts & Crafts Store. Find out more at www.michaels.com

- Visit a pumpkin patch with corn mazes, hayrides, and cider Find one in your area at pumpkinpatchesandmore.org/index.php.

- Go to a "Pick your own" berry, cherry, apple, peach, or pumpkin farm and pick your own fruit

- Attend a free kid's workshop at an Apple retail store to learn more about electronics. www.apple.com/retail/learn/youth

- Attend Home Depot's FREE Kid's workshops held on the first Saturday of every month in all stores from 9am-12:00 (ages 5-12). Children get to keep their craft, plus they receive a certificate of achievement, a Workshop Apron, and a commemorative pin.

- Attend Lowe's Free Kid's Clinic (Build and Grow) held at 10 AM and 2 PM. Check website for exact dates, times, and registration. Each child receives a free apron and goggles, along with their projects and more.

Create!

- Build a tree house or a clubhouse.

- Assemble a model car, ship, or airplane.

- Create whimsical collages or calendars at photomania.net

- Create scrapbooks of your interests, vacations, or special events

- Make a time capsule (be sure to take it with you if you ever move)

- Make a May Day flower basket and then leave it on someone's doorknob or doorstep

- Decorate a pair of flip-flops by hot gluing buttons, jewels or beads on top of the straps

- Make a paper Mache piñata and fill it with small toys or coins instead of candy at parties

- Draw pictures or write out quotes with glow-in-the dark paint then hang the poster on your wall

- Create a dream board collage with pictures and inspirational quotes to motivate you toward your goals

Relax!

- Take a trip to an indoor water park www.indoorwaterpark.net

- Take a trip to a zoo or an aquarium www.aza.org/findzooaquarium

- Solve Sudoku or crossword puzzles

- Search the grass for four-leaf clovers

- Learn to whistle with a blade of grass

- Watch a sunrise or a sunset with a friend
- Wade in a creek and try to catch frogs or crabs
- Make a blanket fort under the dining room table
- Hang a tire swing from a tree in the yard then swing
- Rake up a huge pile of leaves and then jump in them
- Lie in the grass with a friend and share what you see in the cloud formations
- Assemble a jigsaw puzzle and then cover it with clear packing tape and hang it on the wall
- Lie on the grass with a friend at night. Count the stars or find the constellations or look for shooting stars
- Camp in the yard or in the living room with friends during the day or night. Pitch a tent, play a few games, or ask a few questions listed in the "Deepen Your Relationships" section

Get in the Act!

- Enter a Karaoke singing contest
- Make a puppet show stage from a large box and put on a show
- Host a talent show and give a blue ribbon or a small prize to the winner
- Write and act out a play. Build a makeshift stage complete with curtains

- Learn to do magic tricks at www.kidzone.ws/magic/ and then put a show on for family and friends

Throw a Party and Play Games!

Despite all of our media connections, many people feel more disconnected than ever. Play and games are the social oil that lessens the initial friction, to help people become acquainted with and connect to each other.

People also play more passionately when a prize is at stake. Even a dollar trinket will bring out the scholar, jock, or beast in some people. Up the ante with inexpensive rewards such as a small toy, stickers, hair accessories, costume jewelry, or coloring books.

- Plan a surprise birthday party for a friend
- Host a cookout for your friends or neighbors
- Throw a New Year's Eve party and play games
- Throw a St. Patrick's Day party and play games
- Throw a Valentine's Day party and play games
- Have a water-balloon war or distance throwing contest
- Pack a lunch and surprise a friend by going on a picnic
- Host an Easter egg hunt and give small prizes to the winners

- Play *20 Questions, Charades*, *Scrabble* or other board games

- Videos silly antics, fun activities, stunts, mock interviews, or acrobatics

- Hide colored glass beads in the yard and then search for them with flashlights at night

- Take a walk in autumn to collect acorns, horse chestnuts, small evergreen branches, pinecones, and colored leaves to make a festive centerpiece

- Host a real tea party with a pretty teapot and teacups. Dress up in retro clothes and fancy hats. Sip tea with pinkies up.

- Throw a few dollars' worth of change along with a few small toys in a sawdust or confetti pile then let kids dig for buried treasure.

- Have a scavenger hunt or a camera phone scavenger hunt. Make a list of things to find and have the players take pictures of the objects on their cell phones to show that they found the items.

- Have a theme party complete with costumes and decorations such as the Victorian era for a tea party, a 1950s sock hop with poodle skirts and ponytails. Have a Hawaiian luau or a western square dance with cowboys and cowgirls. Plan a Mad Hatter party, or a pirate party with buried treasure, or a sports event with team paraphernalia. Dig through old clothes in the attic or find time period clothes in vintage or thrift stores. Visit partycity.com for more theme party supplies.

The following are a few party games that you may also enjoy.

Ugliest Tie or Sweater Contest – Tell your guests to wear the ugliest tie or sweater they can find when they come to your party. Suggest that they look in their grandparent's attic or a thrift store. Have everyone vote and give the winner a prize.

"Who am I?" – Attach sticky nametags marked with names of famous people, animals, countries, or things in nature on each person's back. (No peeking in mirrors.) Each player can only ask "yes or no" questions. Am I living? Am I a man? Am I a singer? When the person thinks that he knows who or what he is, he asks, "Am I (name)." If he is wrong he keeps playing until he or someone else discovers his or her identity.

The Sandman is best played with a group of eight or more people who are sitting in a circle. A blank slip of paper is placed in a hat or bowl for each player, except for one slip of paper marked with an X. The person who draws the X is the Sandman, who must discretely wink at another person during the course of the game to put them to sleep. When a person sees that a wink is directed at him or her, he or she must announce, "I'm out." The game continues on like this until someone guesses who is putting everyone to sleep.

Steal the Gift – This game is best played with eight or more people. There are three ways to acquire the start-up gifts. One is that the host provides the gently-used "gifts" from his or her belongings. Two is to have each person bring a small wrapped gently-used "gift" from home. The item can be something they no longer want or use, but it should still be in good condition. Gifts can be books, bracelets, candles, small cars, scarves, nail polish, hats, posters, or any other knickknack or bric-a-brac. The third way is to have each player buy a $5 gift, wrap or bag it, and then bring it with them to the party. Here's the setup and the rules:

1. Place all gifts on a table.

2. Have someone write the numbers 1-8 (or however many people are playing) on small slips of paper and then put them in a hat or an opaque bowl.

3. Have each player choose a number.

4. Players sit around the table while one person calls the lowest number.

5. The player with the lowest number chooses a gift and opens it.

6. The next number in sequence is called. This person can either choose a gift from the table or "steal" the other player's opened gift.

7. Every time a gift is stolen from a player, he or she may choose a gift from the table or steal someone else's gift.

8. Continue playing until all the gifts are gone from the table. The gift that you have left at the end of the game is the one that you get to keep.

Prize Ideas for Games: Notepads, activity books, coloring books, crayons, watercolors, markers, safety scissors, glitter pens, sidewalk chalk, puzzles, magazines, bubbles, jump ropes, small cars, plastic cups, hairclips, headbands, bows, lotion, fingernail polish, lip balm, a large bath sponge or puff, Silly Putty, Uno cards, disposable cameras, snow globes, locker mirrors, sun-catchers, window crystals or charms, glow-in-the-dark stars or stickers, glow sticks, nightlights, flashlights.

DEVELOP YOUR INTELLIGENCE

People are naturally drawn to those who have something to share, whether it's fun, educational, exciting, or inspiring. Girls and boys who are involved in projects and activities, whether work or play related, or those who acquire knowledge about many things, are more interesting to be around and possess greater self-confidence. Therefore, they often make friends more easily. Because of this, they form a wider circle of contacts so that when the time comes for dating and marriage they have a greater support system and a larger group of prospects to *choose* from. The wallflower who lacks confidence, or the young adult who has little to discuss because he or she knows little about current events, science, history, or life in general, is usually the one with few friends and few dates or marriage proposals.

Bored people are often BORING people.
Those *who are* INTERESTED in
and **EXCITED** about Life
are usually INTERESTING
and *exciting* people.

We see this happen when a young man or woman is overlooked as a potential companion solely because he or she is boring. Whether teens realize it or not, they intuitively seek companions who are not only attractive and fun, but also fascinating and smart. They seek someone who has ideas to keep life interesting, confidence to keep from seeming needy, knowledge to make wise choices, and a good sense of humor to keep life enjoyable.

It's obvious then that it's not only the outward attraction of physical strength or beauty that wins a heart. It's the well-developed inward strength and beauty of soul that also gains a person's love and affection. Focusing solely on external appearances to attract or to make friends is a shaky base to sustain a relationship. The young man or woman who possesses self-confidence, the teen who is kind and thoughtful, and has a genuine interest in others is the one with magnetic appeal that draws more friends to them.

DO SOMETHING NEW

Someone once said, "The more you learn the more you know. The more you know the smarter you grow. The smarter you grow the louder your voice when speaking your mind or making a choice."

People are instinctively attracted to those who are generous and kind, those who have a happy disposition, a good work ethic, and a positive outlook on life. Two quotes often used when speaking in terms of choosing friends are: "Water seeks its own level," and "Birds of a feather flock together." This is true, but you have the power to choose and to change the depth of your reservoir, or whether you fly with crows or eagles.

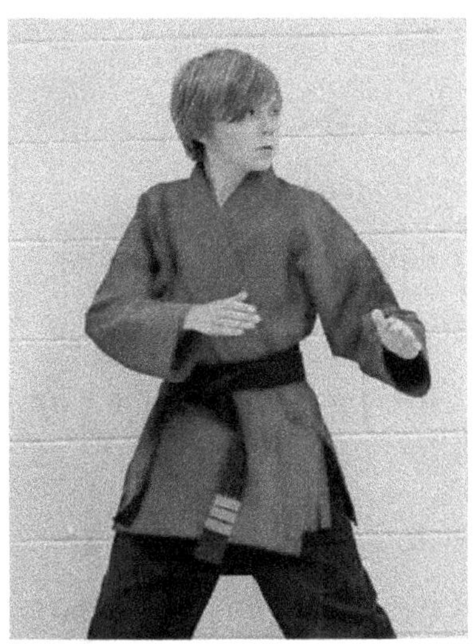

When a person spends a lot of time with someone, or with a particular group of people, he or she often take on similar traits, almost like a chameleon does when it blends in with its surroundings. This is why it's so important to choose your friends wisely and surround yourself with optimistic people, smart people, high-standard people, because someday you may grow to be like them by a process similar to osmosis. You can also try to be a role-model of these quality traits, so others can take their cues from you and be positively influenced for good.

Find someone with similar interests and try a few of the activities mentioned in this book. Who knows? You may develop a friendship that lasts a lifetime.

- Plant a terrarium.
- Take up Tai Chi.
- Take archery lessons.
- Take fencing lessons.
- Plant a flower garden.

- Plant a vegetable garden.
- Learn to knit or crochet.
- Learn a foreign language.
- Learn how to sing or join a choir.
- Learn how to juggle then put on a show.
- Create your own app at www.como.com.
- Learn how to play a musical instrument.
- Learn how to do a professional shoeshine.
- Learn judo, karate, Kung Fu, or kickboxing.
- See our vast universe through a telescope.
- See our miniscule world through a microscope.
- Learn how to sew clothes, curtains, or quilts.
- Learn how to sketch, draw, or paint with acrylics.
- Edit your photos or make a collage at picmonkey.com.
- Create your own website for free at WiX.com or Weebly.com.
- Check out a button maker for your blog at buttongenerator.com.
- Learn to give yourself or someone else a professional manicure.
- Write a song to help you remember long lists or facts for school.
- Plant trees then sell them. Learn how at www.profitableplantsdigest.com/profitable-trees/

- Take a trip to an amusement park. www.themeparkcity.com/WORLD_index.htm
- Find a roller coaster, theme park or thrill ride: www.ultimaterollercoaster.com/themeparks/
- Train for a 5K marathon. Enter and then finish the race with the help of the couch-2-5K running plan.
- Develop your memory by learning all of the Presidents or the books of the Bible or any other long lists in order.
- Create a clickable map for school or to share information and statistics at www.createaclickablemap.com
- Create a blog and share your thoughts, ideas, talents, or experiences with others at www.blogspot.com or wordpress.com
- Take something that you do well and make a step-by-step video on YouTube showing others how to do it. Use a webcam, your cell phone, or use photos for a slideshow presentation.
- Use your own body weight to do resistance exercises such as planks, push-ups, pull-ups, and squats. For the ultimate full body, strength-training, fat-burning exercise, do a few burpees. Burpees are similar to gym class squat-thrusts, but with an added push-up and then jump-up upon rising.

LEARN SOMETHING NEW

Flex and develop your mental muscles by cracking open books, solving puzzles and problems, or by going on new adventures to investigate or invent. Expand your awareness by taking mini-vacations while taking pictures in the process.

Take shots from many angles, perspectives, and distances then create a photo journal. Many interesting sights and sites may be found right in your own hometown.

Every BIG WINNER
was ONCE a BEGINNER
Captain Kangaroo ~ Bob Keeshan

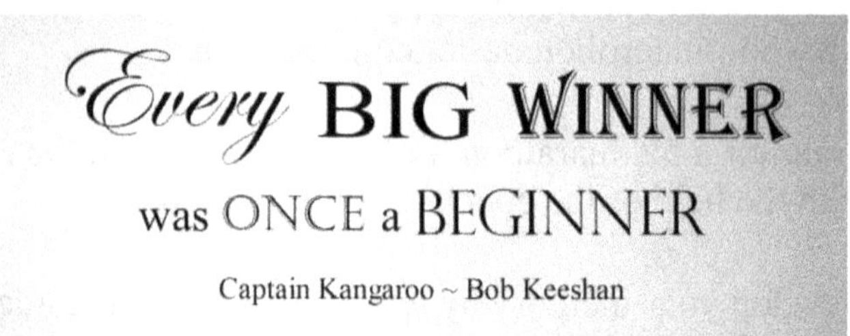

Learn all that you can, all of your life. Material possessions may be lost, stolen or decrease in value, but no one can rob you of the skills, talents, or knowledge that you've acquired, once it's embedded in your brain.

- Visit a fish hatchery.

- Visit a train exhibit or museum.

- Schedule a tour at a fire station in your area.

- Visit a national park in your area. Find one here: www.nps.gov/findapark/index.htm

- Search for art events and exhibits in your area at www.theartguide.com/events

- Get extra help with schoolwork at www.k-12.com.

- Look up information in the National Archives at www.archives.gov.

- Find a radio station anywhere in the world: www.radio-locator.com.

- Take a trip to caves and caverns. For United States visit cavern.com.

- Visit a lighthouse and discover its history then climb the stairs to the top. Find one in your area at: www.unc.edu/~rowlett/lighthouse

- Use the Mindmeister mind-mapping tool to brainstorm and organize your creative ideas at www.mindmeister.com

- Visit museums, living museums, and historic structures in your area. Find one in your area here: www.dir.yahoo.com/arts/humanities/history/u_s__history/living_history/museums_and_memorials

- Visit a Renaissance, Medieval & Pirate Festival. Find one at www.renfaire.com/sites/.

- Learn to write computer HTML code then design your own apps, games and programs at www.code.org.

- Learn to cook healthy food with a creative flair then invite people to try your new recipes.

- Search your local Chamber of Commerce at www.chamberofcommerce.com to find activities and events in your area.

- Learn to identify and use basic hand tools like pliers, screwdrivers, wrenches, and hammers.

- Visit a bookstore and browse around. Ask if any poets or authors will be doing readings or signings.

- Learn everything there is to know about different kinds of animals at www.a-z-animals.com/animals.

- Visit a children's museum of play and interactive exhibits. Find one near you at childrensmuseums.org

- Schedule a field trip to a farm, factory, or a food processing plant. Find one in your area at www.factorytoursusa.com.

- Discover fitness activities, 5K runs, and events in your area at www.active.com or eventbrite.com/directory/sitemap

- Visit a traveling exhibit such as the Vietnam Moving Wall at www.themovingwall.org or the fascinating anatomical Body Worlds at www.bodyworlds.com.

- Get thee to a monastery, cathedral, or basilica and take pictures of the beautiful architecture.

- Watch educational programs on television such as those found on the History Channel, Discovery Channel, Science Channel, National Geographic Channel, or Animal Planet.

- Learn the sounds that birds make and then try to identify them at www.enature.com/birding/audio.asp.

- Challenge yourself at an Outward Bound Leadership Program: www.outwardbound.org.

- Read the calendar of events listed in your local newspaper, or check events guides: www.usa.worldweb.com/Events/.

- Check out tourism directories published by your state or county. www.usa.gov/Citizen/Topics/Travel-Tourism/State-Tourism.shtml

- Search Google books to see if anyone has written about your family genealogy. Use keywords such as your mother's maiden name, places where your grandparents were born, or places family members have ever lived.

- Take a pocket field guide or look over one online here: www.enature.com/fieldguides, and then go for a walk in the woods to learn the names of birds, bugs, bees, leaves, trees, or flowers.

- Take a hike in the woods and listen to the sounds of nature. Focus on the surroundings. Smell the scents and feel the textures in the area. Notice how many sights and sounds are different from the city.

- Check out *Scigirls* on television or online and watch the girls do experiments: www.pbskids.org/scigirls/index

- Visit a botanical garden. Take pictures and learn the names of flowers and plants.

- Visit a science, history or art museum. Find one at www.museumspot.com/categories/science.htm. Choose your state or your country from the categories on the left side of the webpage then refine your search from there.

- Check out *Fetch! Ruff Ruffman*, a fun science program on television or online, to see experiments and how things work. www.pbskids.org/fetch/games/index.html.

- Visit a college or local library to look up events in the newspaper archives. You can also check out online archives at www.newspapers.com / www.freenewspaperarchives.us/

- Visit a library, not only to take out books, but also to check out the activities they have to offer. Most small libraries have a children's holiday or summer reading programs, craft hours, story hours, or a room where you can research local history.

- Visit waterfalls and gorges in your area. www.gowaterfalling.com/index.shtml.

- Check out the tourism guide for your state here www.sidestreet.com/usatourism/. A worldwide directory can be found at www.placesbook.org/

- Take apart a broken alarm clock, mixer, or lamp to see how it works and then put it back together again. (Be sure that the appliance is unplugged before you begin.) Draw diagrams of the parts and placements as you take it apart to help you remember how to reassemble it again.

- Research your local history. Find out if any significant events occurred in your hometown. See if any famous people were born where you live. Visit landmarks, monuments, or notable places of historical interest. Visit your local Chamber of Commerce and pick up informative brochures. Put together a walking tour of your city and then take out-of-town family and friends on a tour. Take a friend or a date on a site-seeing tour of your city. Pretend you're tourists and take lots of pictures. Google or find out more at your local library, historical society, or at www.preservationdirectory.com.

- Apply to Boys and Girls State where each participant learns about government and love of God and country as they spend an intensive week of developing leadership skills and studying government. In many cases, most expenses associated with attending this program are sponsored by an American Legion Post, a local business or another community-based organization.

  Boys and girls must be entering their senior year of high school to be eligible. The American Legion Boys and Girls State is among the most respected educational programs of government instruction for high school students. Many are also eligible to earn three college credits. Find out more at www.boysandgirlsstate.org

READ TO FEED YOUR BRAIN

You've heard the old saying, "You are what you eat," but the same holds true that you are what you think. And what you think is influenced by what you read, what you see, and what you hear, especially through books, movies, music, and other forms of media. Just as a steady diet of junk food harms a healthy body, a steady diet of inferior media harms a healthy mind.

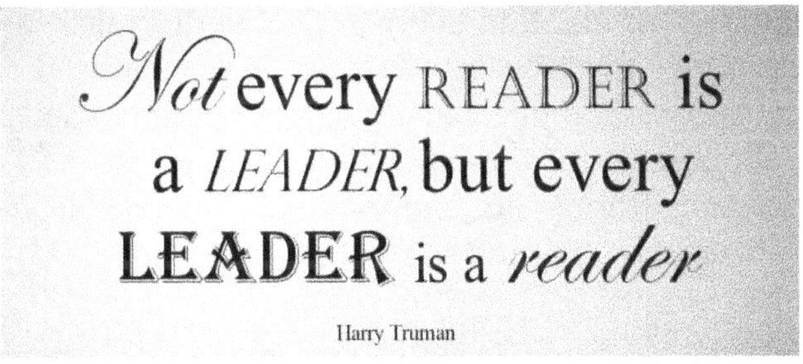

What you feed your mind is either healthy food for thought or junk food for the brain, and it determines whether you are spiritually, mentally, and physically fit or frail.

People often chant, "Read! Read! Read, to become a better person," but there are many books in the world that do nothing to stimulate intellectual or creative growth or promote healthy thinking. It's up to you to choose what is best for you. James Allen wrote in his classic book, *As a Man Thinketh*:

> "A man's mind may be likened to a garden, which may be intelligently cultivated or allowed to run wild; but whether cultivated or neglected, it must, and will, bring forth. If no useful seeds are put into it, then an abundance of useless weed-seeds will fall therein, and will continue to produce their kind."

There's a slew of mental junk food being served up in the world today, and it's often just as difficult to correct a child's mental diet as it is to correct their physical diet. Yet we need to weed out the unwholesome books and media that influence their minds and choke out healthy thinking. Books and movies should not only entertain, but also help children learn to discern what is right and wrong, true and false, or that which inspires or drags down.

Reading to your children every single day or night is one of the best things that you can do to give them a head start on learning and develop their intelligence. Fill their shelves with books about nature and animals, mystery and science, novels of love and stories of triumph, along with inspirational biographies and other true stories.

One way to prepare preschoolers for reading is to play word games with them. Ask them to think of as many words as they can that rhyme with a word that you give them. Do the same for opposites. Ask them what sounds various animals make. Tell them stories from your childhood by retelling them in a story-like fashion. Tell them about your pets or where you lived while you were growing up. These concept games and stories can be played or shared in the evening to help them wind-down before bed.

Avid reading increases a child's comprehension to help him or her learn more in school and in everyday life. A voracious reader often becomes a better writer and a more eloquent speaker. It's a sad fact that no matter how smart people are, others will often judge their level of intelligence by how well they speak and whether they are articulate or tongue-tied or use slang or crude language. Reading seems to bring the positive qualities of speech and expression about by osmosis after "hearing" the author's voice through the written words.

Audio books and books on CD are easy ways to get kids reading too. Pop in a CD while driving in the car and they can follow along in the book. If a child is ill in bed or visually impaired, audio books can help break up the boredom. You can also find many children's books on major online bookstores or at www.Audible.com. Many digital books are free through local and county library systems. Children with reading disabilities may also be eligible for free digital downloads. Ask the child's school librarian or special education department for help in facilitating registration.

Encourage children to read biographies about men and women who have overcome hardships and adversity. A few of the people who have inspired multitudes by their examples are Jesus Christ, Harriet Tubman, Booker T. Washington, George Washington Carver, Florence Nightingale, Abraham Lincoln, Orville and Wilber Wright, Henry Ford, Thomas Edison, Annie Sullivan, and Mahatma Gandhi. Most of these men and women are mentioned in history books, but their humble beginnings are often omitted. Investigate and discover the fascinating struggles that they endured before reaching their places of prominence.

Encourage children to read fiction that teaches the consequences of making poor choices and the advantages of making wise choices such as those found in Aesop's Fables, especially "The Tortoise and the Hare," "The Miller, the Boy, and the Donkey," and "The Crow and the Cheese."

There are thousands of great books in the world today, but I'm only mentioning a few to get your own memory stream flowing. What were your favorite books when you were a child? Chances are they are books that your children will enjoy reading today. Expand the brain not the body. Read! Read! Read! Rah! Rah! Rah!

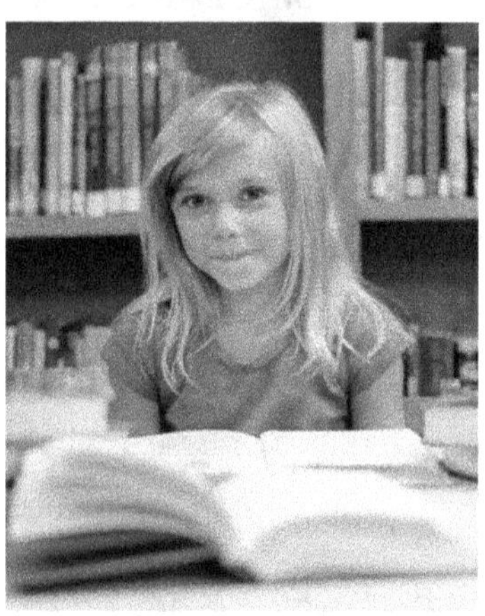

Non-fiction Short Stories for Younger Children

Step into Reading books contain fascinating stories about people, places, events, and animals, to entertain and educate a child and to encourage a lifelong love of learning. The following books are geared toward children 4 through 9 years old. Some of the stories may spark a child's interest enough, where they may want to do further research.

- *Abe Lincoln's Hat:* President Lincoln was often forgetful so he solved this problem by storing important papers in his top hat!

- *Baseball's Best: Five True Stories:* Hall of Fame legends, Babe Ruth, Joe DiMaggio, Jackie Robinson, Roberto Clemente, and Hank Aaron.

- *Ben Franklin and the Magic Squares:* Ben Franklin's magic square is a box of nine numbers arranged so that any line of three numbers adds up to the same number.

- *Christopher Columbus:* The sailors' fears and Columbus's courage, along with information about the journey, old maps (compared to current ones), and a cutaway view of the ship make this book an informative and interesting read.

- *Dinosaur Days:* Children follow a day in the life of Triceratops and his scary encounter with a Tyrannosaurus Rex.

- *Discovery in the Cave:* An amazing true adventure story about children discovering the Lascaux Cave prehistoric paintings.

- *DK Eyewitness Books:* These books are loaded with beautiful photos and relevant information pertaining to history, science, people, places, and things.

- *DK Eyewitness Classics:* Literature in a condensed easy-to-read book with illustrations and photographs.

- *Eat My Dust! Henry Ford's First Race:* In 1901, Henry Ford needed money to build cars so other people could afford them, so he enters a car race to raise the money.

- *Escape North! The Story of Harriet Tubman:* From child slave to a conductor on the Underground Railroad to a fighter for equal rights and a spy in the Civil War, Harriet Tubman is one of America's greatest female role models in history.

- *Francis Scott Key's Star-Spangled Banner:* After the battle at Fort McHenry, Francis was inspired by what he saw, so he wrote a poem that would become America's national anthem.

- *George Washington and the General's Dog:* While George Washington is fighting in the American Revolution, he saw a lost dog on the battlefield then showed kindness and courage in returning the dog to its owner.

- *Ice Mummy:* Two tourists hiking in the Alps found a man who had been frozen in the ice for 5,000 years.

- *Lewis and Clark: A Prairie Dog for the President:* In 1803, President Thomas Jefferson sends Lewis and Clark out west to explore, to make maps, to draw pictures, and to collect plants. He also asks them to send presents back to him.

- *Listen Up!: Alexander Graham Bell's Talking Machine:* Alexander Graham Bell goes to the World's Fair to show off his new talking machine, but he's unsure if anyone will come to see it or if the telephone will even work.

- *Looking for Bigfoot:* Learn about the legendary Sasquatch. Is it a myth or is it real?

- *Moonwalk: The First Trip:* Learn about Apollo II's historic flight, lift-off, splashdown, and quarantine.

- *Pompeii...Buried Alive!* Learn about the village of Pompeii and how its people were buried alive when Mount Vesuvius erupted 2,000 years ago.

- *The Bravest Dog Ever: The True Story of Balto:* The true story about a sled dog who led his team through snow and ice over 50 miles of northern Alaska wilderness to deliver medicine during an epidemic.

- *The First Thanksgiving:* A vivid account of the Pilgrims' journey, struggles, and Thanksgiving celebration in easy-to-read language.

- *The Great Houdini:* Harry Houdini was poor as a child, but he worked very hard to eventually become the greatest escape artist of all time.

- *The Titanic: Lost and Found:* Follow this exciting yet tragic account of the world's most famous disaster-at-sea and the discovery of the Titanic remains many years later.

- *The Trojan Horse: How the Greeks Won the War* Discover how the Greeks tricked the Trojans and rescued Helen of Troy.

- *To the Top! Climbing the World's Highest Mountain*: An exciting story about the climb of a lifetime up Mount Everest, while fighting perilous snow, ice, and wind, while knowing that 19 others had died in the same attempt.

- *Trail of Tears:* The tragic story of how settlers moving west forced the Cherokee Nation to leave their homeland and travel over 1,000 miles to Oklahoma.

- *True Life Treasure Hunts:* A story about a real pirate's lost treasure and how it was discovered 300 years later.

Periodical Paradise

Subscribe to magazines that interest your children. If your kids are reading them they're still *reading* and *learning* as long as they're quality periodicals. Check out some of these amazing, trustworthy, and award-winning magazines to pique your child's interest and to develop a love affair with reading. Some of the subscriptions may be a bit pricey, but the articles, stories and activities will supply your child with positive and educational alternatives to video games and social media.

Adventures in Odyssey

American Girl

Cat Fancy

Clubhouse / Clubhouse Jr.

Cobblestone

Cricket

Dog Fancy

Highlights for Children

Horse Illustrated

Humpty Dumpty

Jack and Jill

Kid's Discover

Keys for Kids Daily Devotional (Free)

National Geographic for Kids

Odyssey

Ranger Rick

Sports Illustrated for Kids

Turtle

Young Rider

Zoobooks

Go for the Gold!

One of the reasons English majors study great works of literature is because human nature basically stays the same throughout the ages, and eternal truths never grow old. Many of the following classic works are also available as DVDs, but I would encourage children to read the books, to exercise their minds and to gain greater depth of understanding, since the characters' thoughts are difficult to portray on screen.

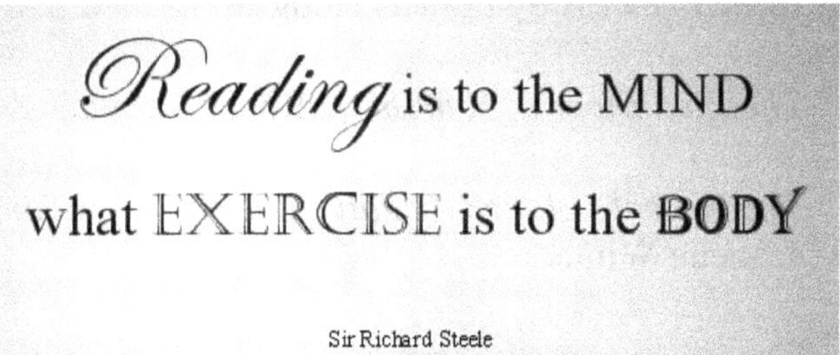

Most of these golden oldies (and newer classics) can be found in libraries or online, or if you wish, as movies to buy, borrow, or rent. Although some movies may be difficult to find, the messages are worth the time and detective work in finding them. Some of the classics come in easy-to-read versions, but obviously you can choose the more in-depth version for older children. Many of these classics are free or very affordable in eBook format. Of course, there are many, many more great books than the ones I have listed here.

Younger Children

- *Aesop's Fables*

- *Heidi* by Johanna Spyri

- Children's Bible Stories

- *Owl at Home* by Arnold Lobel

- *Frog and Toad* by Arnold Lobel

- *Madeline* by Ludwig Bemelmans

- *The Gruffalo* by Julia Donaldson

- *Ferdinand the Bull* by Munro Leaf

- *Little Princess* by Francis Hodgson Bernett

- *The Pied Piper of Hamlin* by Robert Browning

- *The Watcher: Jane Goodall's Life with the Chimps* by Jeanette Winter

- The Classic Starts Series (50+ titles) is easy to read and age appropriate, yet respects the original work.

Older Children

- *Black Beauty* by Anna Sewell

- *Christy* by Catherine Marshall
- *Moby Dick* by Herman Melville
- *As a Man Thinketh* by James Allen
- *Pride and Prejudice* by Jane Austin
- *Lord of the Rings* by J. R. R. Tolkien
- *Little Women* by Louisa May Alcott
- *The Jungle Book* by Rudyard Kipling
- *A Christmas Carol* by Charles Dickens
- *The Odyssey* by Homer / Robert Fagles
- *The Death of Ivan Ilych* by Leo Tolstoy
- *Uncle Tom's Cabin* by Harriet Beecher Stowe
- *The Greatest Thing in the World* by Henry Drummond
- *Ann of Green Gables Collection* by Lucy Laud Montgomery
- *The Adventures of Sherlock Holmes* by Arthur Conan Doyle
- *The Lion the Witch and the Wardrobe* and other books by C.S. Lewis

- *Chicken Soup for the Soul* books by Jack Canfield, Mark Victor Hansen and contributing authors

- *The Holy Bible*: Examples, stories and teachings about love, courage, faith, guidance, advice, poetry, and parables.

Overcoming Life's Hurdles

The following true stories in books or DVDs are inspiring examples of how faith and perseverance helped these underdogs overcome obstacles and succeed in reaching their goals in life. A man name Forbes said, "History has demonstrated that the most notable winners usually encountered heartbreaking obstacles before they triumphed. They won because they refused to become discouraged by their defeats."

DVDs

- *Rudy* (for football fans)

- *Miracle* (for hockey fans)

- *Pride* (for swim team fans)

- *Hoosiers* (for basketball fans)

- *The Rookie* (for baseball fans)

- *We are Marshall* (for football fans)

- *Glory Road* (for college basketball fans)

- *Unconditional* (helping inner-city children)

- *The Miracle Worker* (overcoming disabilities)
- *The Greatest Game Ever Played* (for golf fans)
- *Spartacus* (for history fans - Kirk Douglas version)
- *Stand and Deliver* (outstanding academic achievement)
- *The King's Speech* (King George VI's quest to overcome his speech impediment)

Books

- *Love Lucy* by Lucille Ball
- *Out of the Depths* by John Newton
- *The Story of my Life* by Helen Keller
- *Up From Slavery* by Booker T. Washington
- *George Muller of Bristol* by Arthur T. Pierson
- *Wilma Rudolph: Olympic Runner* by Jo Harper
- *American Miler: The Life and Times of Glenn Cunningham* by Paul J. Kiell
- *The Perfect Mile: Three Athletes, One Goal, and Less Than Four Minutes to Achieve It* by Neal Bascomb
- *A Narrative of the Life of Mary Jemison: the White Woman of the Genesee* by W.P. Letchworth

DIM THE LIGHTS FOR MOVIE NIGHT

Just as reading has a huge impact on life, so does what we see and hear. The eyes and ears are the doorways through which information enters the heart. Movies often contain blatant or subliminal messages that leave imprints on impressionable hearts and minds. The following true stories, old classics, and inspiring and thought-provoking movies will not only entertain, but also educate and enlighten, as they show glimpses of history and insights into humanity.

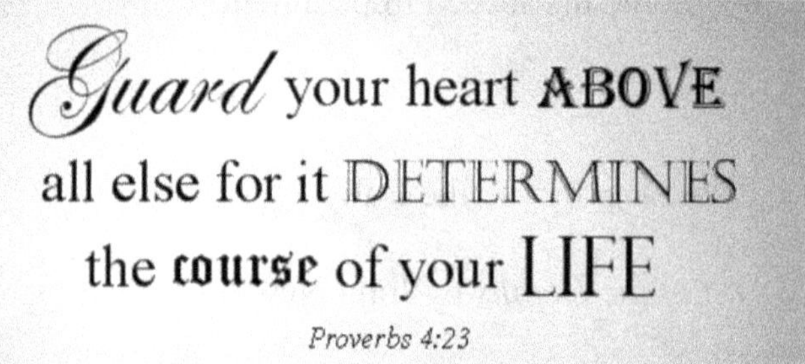

Many of these movies, though seemingly old-fashioned, are based on the wisdom of timeless truths. A few of the movies are autobiographical or based on true stories. Others are works of fiction, but still inspirational or fun nonetheless. Make movie night a special event with pillows and popcorn and non-sugary drinks. Assemble your brood, light a few candles, and turn off the lights then enjoy a time of togetherness. You may also need a box of tissues since some of these movies are real tear-jerkers.

- *A Walk to Remember*
- *Andre*
- *Annie*
- *Babe*
- *Ben Hur*

- *Charlotte's Web*
- *Diary of Anne Frank*
- *Dr. Quinn Medicine Woman series*
- *Facing the Giants*
- *Fly Away Home*
- *Flywheel*
- *Gone With the Wind*
- *Hachi: A Dog's Tale*
- *Harvey*
- *It's a Wonderful Life*
- *Lilies of the Field*
- *Little House on the Prairie Series*
- *Lonesome Dove Series*
- *Mary Poppins*
- *Mighty Joe Young*
- *Mr. Holland's Opus*
- *My Fair Lady*
- *Old Yeller*
- *Pollyanna*
- *Pride and Prejudice*
- *Roman Holiday*
- *Roots*
- *Schindler's List*

- *Sense and Sensibility*
- *Swiss Family Robinson*
- *The Buttercream Gang*
- *The Sound of Music*
- *The Trouble with Angels*
- *To Sir with Love*
- *White Fang*

You can also prescreen DVDs and movies by reading reviews at www.pluggedin.com or www.kids-in-mind.com. These sites offer detailed synopsizes concerning movie content to inform the viewer as to how much drinking, smoking, swearing, or violence is in the movie, or how many drug, sexual, or anti-religious comments or situations are contained in each movie.

DEEPEN YOUR RELATIONSHIPS

When I was fifteen years-old, I went to the lake with a group of my friends and then decided to go into the water while they stayed on the beach. I didn't know how to swim very well, but I knew how to float on my back, so I foolishly assumed that I would be okay. After a few moments of drifting atop the gentle waves, I stepped down, but barely touched the sand with the tip of my toe, so I panicked. And then I bounced. Up and down, on my toe, while lifting my chin as high as I could and raising my hand in the air. On the third bounce, my friend saw that I was in distress. Mimi quickly jumped into the lake and brought me safely to the shore. Even though I never went completely under water, I believe that without her help this could have been a tragic situation.

My friend was not only "there for me," but she took action when it was needed. Back on the beach, we went about our business like nothing had ever happened. We didn't talk about it, report it, or analyze it. She didn't boast about her rescue, or reprimand me for making an unwise move. And we never brought the incident up again until later on in life.

> *"If only* someone WOULD **LISTEN** to ME."
>
> Job 31:35, Holy Bible

People need a trusted friend when they're on the throes of drowning. A listening ear to hear without condemnation. Someone who loves them enough to teach them to swim, or to pull them back to solid ground when they are struggling to keep their head above water or to merely stay afloat.

THE BUDDY SYSTEM

The following questions are divided into three sections that move from shallow to deep levels of communication. Some of the questions are meant to be fun, while others have the potential to deepen existing relationships or mend those in need of support or repair. Many of the questions are frivolous and silly, while others are more thought-provoking and may even provide a measure of emotional healing.

The latter questions may also help those who feel overwhelmed to keep them from drowning in anger, frustration or feelings of hopelessness. If you plan to work through this list with a friend, family member, or significant other, the questions should be asked in the *group order* listed in order to build trust. Some of the "Wading off Shore" questions can be asked to younger children for fun without continuing on into the deeper waters. If the child feels uncomfortable answering any these questions, he or she can set out on a solo voyage of self-discovery with pen and pad in hand to answer these questions alone.

The "game" begins as a silly quiz or interview, but gradually becomes more in-depth with the purpose of helping the child or adult become more open and self-aware. This insight allows the person to emerge and grow toward his or her fullest potential.

I encourage you to ask only a few questions at a time, but then ask one or two more questions in addition to the original one, such as, "How did (does) that make you feel?" or "What can you do about it?" or "What is it about that one that you like so much?" to keep the conversation rolling.

This open dialogue can strengthen family connections or tighten bonds that are already in place with a friend. This interview is meant to be played with *both* people taking turns, asking questions, and exchanging answers, so there will be *equal sharing time* for each person. This shared knowledge provides leverage to those who have dared to open their hearts and expose their thoughts, dreams, and even their wounds, since the other person has also done the same.

This shared information also helps ensure that there will be no emotional harm done via gossip or online social chitchat, since both participants are making themselves open and vulnerable. When this deep level of camaraderie is established, the friendship often becomes stronger. This mutual unity creates a protective wall to shield, support, and guide those involved, as they venture out into an ever-changing and oftentimes harsh or confusing world.

Are you ready? Here we go…

WADING OFF SHORE

In this section, the conversation begins with causal questions that lay the foundation of trust. Wading off shore is a safe way to test the waters before playing in the deeper waves. If the answers to these shallow questions are met with anything but utmost acceptance, the person will learn not to reveal deeper thoughts in the future.

1. What is your favorite flower?
2. What is your favorite movie?
3. What is your favorite smell?
4. Who or what makes you smile?
5. Have you ever had a nickname?
6. What song best describes your life?
7. What person do you admire the most?
8. What is your favorite outdoor activity?
9. What is your favorite month or season?
10. What is the best book you've ever read?
11. What is your earliest childhood memory?
12. Have you ever won a contest or an award?
13. What does your dream vacation look like?
14. If you were an animal, what would you be?
15. Have you ever broken a bone or had stitches?
16. What is the first thing you notice about a person?
17. What is the most beautiful sight you have ever seen?

18. If you were a car or a truck, what kind would you be?

19. Which school teacher do you remember the most? Why?

20. If you could go anywhere in the world, where would you go?

21. Who is the most famous person you have ever seen or met?

22. If you had one wish what would it be? (Besides more wishes.)

23. What is the most memorable scene from your favorite movie?

24. Who has made you laugh more than anyone else? Describe a situation.

25. What was your first impression of me? (The person asking the questions.)

26. What is the funniest thing that has ever happened to you or to someone you know?

27. If you could spend one day with a famous person from the past or present, who would it be?

28. If your house caught on fire, what would you grab as you ran out the door (besides a person or pet)?

29. If you were stranded on a deserted island, what is one thing that you would want to have with you?

30. If someone wanted to make a movie about your life, what actor do you feel would best play your part?

PLAYING IN THE WAVES

As this interview "game" progresses, the person asking the questions should make a vow of confidentiality to ensure trust. The promise should sound something like this: "I want you to know that you mean a lot to me, and you can talk to me about anything. No matter what you tell me, whether good or bad, I will always love you, and I will never share what you say with anyone else, without your permission."

Your verbal guarantee gives the person courage to speak freely. This openness of thoughts and feelings may also help the child or adult emotionally heal, if needed. Floating on the waves is an easy way to become accustomed to deeper water. These questions are a bit more personal, but many are still breezy and fun. The same rules apply.

31. What is your pet peeve?

32. What do you dread doing?

33. What is your favorite quote?

34. What is your greatest strength?

35. What is your favorite love song?

36. What do you believe about God?

37. What do you believe about angels?

38. What is your definition of success?

39. Who do you look up to as a role model?

40. What book has influenced you the most?

41. What is your fondest childhood memory?

42. What is your most embarrassing moment?

43. When have you felt the most safe and secure?

44. What do you think about when you daydream?

45. What mistake or hardship taught you a lesson?

46. When do you feel the most alive or energized?

47. What song makes you happy when you hear it?

48. What is one word that describes your personality?

49. What would you be happy doing for hours on end?

50. What would you do if you knew you couldn't fail?

51. What do you admire about your mother or your father?

52. What is the most daring thing that you have ever done?

53. What legacy would you like to leave after you are gone?

54. What is the craziest thing that you have ever seen someone do?

55. What are the most meaningful words that you have ever heard?

56. If you could accomplish anything in the world, what would it be?

57. If someone wrote a book about your life, what would the title be?

58. What is the one thing you know you'll regret, if you never get to do it?

59. If you could change anything about yourself or your life, what would it be?

60. What quality do you possess that you hope your children will someday possess?

61. If you were going to lose one of your senses, and you had the ability to choose which one, what would it be?

62. What would you give to a special friend (as a gift), if you could only give them your time, talent, or something you own?

SWIMMING IN THE DEEP

When swimmers feel secure after playing in the waves, they may be more inclined to venture into the deep, if a faithful friend is there for support or to teach them how to swim. The simple question of "How did that make you feel?" often has the potential to open a flow of emotions that have been buried in the deep.

When this emotional gate is open, it is best to be shockproof and just listen, or ask a few non-intrusive questions without offering advice. If you show any sign of sudden surprise, or offer unheeded counsel during a sensitive or hot topic, the gate often slams shut and the conversation ends.

When a child or adult feels free to reveal his or her heart to another person, their words often become the catharsis that siphons off hot or toxic emotions, so healing and restoration can begin. If the unhealthy emotions happen to be directed toward you, it is best to just sit and listen while nodding in agreement with an attitude of acceptance, until the person has finished venting. Defending yourself at this point will also shut the gate and the conversation will end (or flare up).

Your silence does not necessarily mean that the child or adult is right and you are wrong. You are merely acknowledging and respecting his or her right to *feel* as they do. When the person has finished speaking, you may need to ask for clarification or forgiveness, and then ask what you can do to fix the offense or improve the situation. And then by all means, do your best to make amends and take the steps to restore the relationship. Once this has been completed, a floodgate of positive and healthy emotions often begin to emerge.

When you begin this level of swimming in the deep, it's best to set the stage. Profound questions are often easier to answer when a friend or family member is facing *the same direction* as the person asking the questions, such as while sitting on a porch, deck, or patio loveseat in the evening by moonlight, candlelight, or solar lights; or while sitting side-by-side in front of a fire-pit or campfire; or while riding together in a car on a road-trip, especially in the evening.

A similar scenario can be arranged on a park or piano bench, or while washing and rinsing dishes together. There seems to be less intimidation in answering personal questions when both people are facing the same direction, particularly in subdued lighting.

If you are trustworthy, shockproof, and non-judgmental, a person will tell you almost anything. Ask questions that will help them find answers, rather than voice your opinion, unless, of course, they ask for it. The following questions have the potential to evoke an array of emotions ranging from laughter to tears. Therefore, the one asking the questions should also be prepared to listen with empathy and sympathy, along with confidentiality.

You may also want to rephrase the person's answer back to him or her in a gentle tone of voice to let them know that they've been heard. This is similar to what drive-thru restaurant servers do when they repeat your order back to you. This paraphrasing also confirms that you understood what they said.

For example, Sally says, "I felt like I was invisible." Joan then *softly* says, "You must have felt so all alone." Instantly, Sally feels understood and the emotional gate inside her heart opens up a little bit more.

The reflective response reassures Sally that she has been heard, and it helps her feel safe and accepted. As a result, she is more inclined to continue sharing her thoughts and emotions as the conversation continues.

A few casual questions are interspersed with the serious ones to give the swimmers time to exhale.

Ready? Take a deep breath.

63. When have you felt the *most* loved?

64. What was a pivotal point in your life?

65. When was the happiest day of your life?

66. When was the saddest day of your life?

67. What is your greatest accomplishment?

68. What is your biggest regret?

69. What is one struggle that you have overcome?

70. What is one struggle that you have yet to overcome?

71. If you could do anything in your life over again, what would it be?

72. What popular idea do you think the world has wrong?

73. Who has inspired you to become a better person?

74. What do you believe about the afterlife?

75. Who is the most courageous person you know or have ever heard about in history?

76. What do you hope to accomplish in your life?

77. What would you like written on your tombstone someday?

78. What do you wish you could say to someone who has hurt you?

79. What do you wish someone who has hurt you, would say to you?

80. What is the kindest thing that anyone has ever done for you?

81. What is the kindest thing that you have ever done for someone else?

82. What has someone done that made you love them more?

83. What has someone done that made you respect them more?

84. Have you ever wanted to run away?

85. If you could bring someone you know back into your life for one day, who would it be, and what would you say to him or her?

86. What is something you would love to do but lack the courage to do it?

87. Who do you find hard to forgive?

88. What do you believe is the most important thing in life?

89. What song makes you feel sad when you hear it?

90. What do you feel that you do well?

91. How do you know I love you?

92. What is the hardest thing you've ever done?

93. What is the scariest thing you've ever experienced?

94. If you had twenty-four hours to live, what would you do?

95. What three people have made a difference in your life?

96. What is the most important thing you would like to do before you die?

97. What would you do if you weren't afraid?

98. What makes you feel the most loved?

Wouldn't you feel valued or cherished if someone took the time to ask you these questions and then listened to your answers with heartfelt interest and empathy?

A bond is not only formed between the person asking the questions and the person answering them, but studies have also shown that emotional healing often takes place when someone feels that he or she is completely *heard, understood,* and *unconditionally accepted* by at least *one* person. One person! Amazing.

Overall health and mental health thrive in this type of environment and healing often spills over into the physical realm too, once the soul is opened, loved, and protected under this cloak of camaraderie.

LIFE PRESERVERS

Years ago, there was a show on television called *The $64,000 Question.* The game was played like many of today's competitive shows, where the questions become more difficult as the contestants progress to the next level.

While $64,000 may not seem like a lot of money compared to shows like *Who Wants to be a Millionaire*, it was a lot of loot back in the 1950s. Answering all the questions correct had the potential to drastically change the player's life.

The following question will not necessarily make you rich, although it quite possibly could in the future, but it is meant to discover where your passion lies, to buoy your life and other people's lives for good. This passion has the potential to make you rich *inside,* as you *enrich the lives of others*. These meaningful deeds deposit true wealth internally and eternally.

The $64,000 Question

> What is something you love to do, something you could do for hours on end, even if you weren't getting paid for it, but felt that by giving your service away it would *benefit other people*?

Simply put, what makes your heart go pitter-patter? What lights your inner fire of desire when you think about making a difference in the world? Once you have the answer, ask yourself: ***What is the first step I need to take to begin moving in this direction?***
The answer to this question has the potential to become a life-changer for you, and a life-preserver for other people.

In order to live a meaningful life, you must do meaningful deeds. Take the plunge!

DEDICATE YOUR TIME

One of life's paradoxes is that when we help other people, we indirectly help ourselves. Children should be encouraged to do volunteer work, or to give of themselves in some other charitable way, and in doing so they will be helping themselves to become better friends, neighbors, and citizens. This volunteer work should be above and beyond what is required for school, club memberships, or potential scholarships.

The Golden Rule

So in EVERYTHING, do to **OTHERS** what you would have them do **TO YOU**.

Jesus Christ

Volunteer work will not only benefit others, but it will also provide children with a feeling of fulfillment and a sense of purpose and meaning as they make a difference in someone else's life. Service should neither be done for recognition, nor for pay, but for the sole satisfaction that grows on the inside and emerges as a smile on the outside. This feeling of purpose and meaning also has the potential to attract friends and other wonderful things to the child. This is because service also builds confidence and establishes a good reputation. It instills a feeling of self-worth and teaches one of the most fundamental spiritual and natural laws, which is that of sowing and reaping. It also keeps them from becoming self-absorbed.

Acts of kindness also produce feelings of inner-satisfaction, which in turn may also reduce episodes of emotional or escape eating. Face-to-face and heart-to-heart exchanges often reduce hand-to-mouth exchanges of food.

Most of these projects can be done alone, but some of them are easier and more fun to do with a group of friends. If a child doesn't know what a person needs, he or she can just ask the simple question: "What can I do to help you?" After volunteering in the community, children can eventually think about working on a wider scale throughout their lives to make a difference in their county, state, country, and world.

VOLUNTEER YOUR TIME, ENERGY, AND TALENT

Volunteer your time, energy, and talents on young and old alike, by showing them kindness and by helping them with things they may struggle with on their own, or things they cannot do for themselves. Get a group of friends together to assist the elderly or disabled. Offer to help them with home repairs, yard work, errands, and odd jobs. Service should be offered with the sole intent of helping someone without any expectations.

- Volunteer to rake leaves.

- Volunteer to wash a car.

- Volunteer to run an errand.

- Volunteer to mow the lawn.
- Volunteer to wash windows.
- Organize a car wash fundraiser.
- Volunteer to paint for someone.
- Volunteer as a junior fire fighter.
- Volunteer to tutor kids in your school.
- Volunteer to pull weeds from a garden.
- Volunteer to brush the snow from a car.
- Volunteer to answer phones at a telethon.
- Volunteer for a mission's trip through a church.
- Volunteer to deliver flowers to patients at a hospital.
- Volunteer to shovel snow from a sidewalk or driveway.
- Volunteer to collect for UNICEF at www.unicefusa.org.
- Collect clothes and blankets to donate to a homeless shelter.
- Volunteer to read to someone who is ill, blind, or bedridden.
- Volunteer to help save the whales at www.savethewhales.org.

- Build a float for a parade to raise awareness for a worthy cause.

- Volunteer to become a Big Brother or a Big Sister at www.bbbs.org.

- Volunteer or donate to the Kids in Need Foundation at www.kinf.org.

- Volunteer at a local soup kitchen, food pantry, or food gleaning program.

- Volunteer at Habitat for Humanity to help build a home at www.habitat.org.

- Volunteer for the Meals on Wheels program in your area at www.mowaa.org.

- Collect and distribute hats, gloves, and umbrellas too underprivileged children.

- Volunteer to sing or play an instrument at a church or a senior housing complex.

- Organize a benefit to get school supplies into the hands of underprivileged children.

- Find an area of interest where you would like to volunteer at www.volunteermatch.org.

- Matte or frame artwork or photographs and sell them. Donate the proceeds to a worthy cause.

- Volunteer to help out at your local SPCA, humane society, shelter, or animal rescue group at www.spcai.org.

- Volunteer to host a fundraiser or math-a-thon for St. Jude's Children's Research Hospital at stjude.org.

- Create a personalized calendar to sell as a fundraiser. Use photos of firemen, policemen, doctors, teachers, or anyone else who has made a difference in other people's lives: www.calendarfundraising.com

- Join forces with other health conscious people and create a cookbook of nutritious foods to sell and raise money for cancer research or some other worthy cause: www.morriscookbooks.com

- Answer fun and educational questions while accumulating ten grains of rice for each correct answer at www.freerice.com. All collected rice will be donated to feed hungry people. (Be sure to sign in each time you begin.)

- Arrange a 5K Benefit Walk for someone who is recovering from the loss of their home due to wind, water, quake, or fire, or any other natural disaster.

- Collect non-perishable food and donate it to women's shelter, homeless shelter, food bank, or soup kitchen.

- Obtain permission to use an abandoned house or building and then create a setting that represents your cause. Recruit people to become actors and have them dress the part to raise awareness of thc situation. Ask the public for prop donations to furnish the scene. Do the homework and make each scene as realistic as possible. Charge admission as each spectator moves amid the setting. Donate the proceeds to your cause.

NO ALLOWANCE ALLOWED

Children should not be given an allowance lest they acquire a sense of entitlement later on in life. It also stifles motivation and creativity. I'm not referring to gifts or special events, but rather a predictable weekly allowance of money for doing absolutely nothing. When my daughters were teens and wanted an allowance, I couldn't afford to shell out money for them to spend frivolously, so I offered to pay them minimum wage instead, for doing small jobs around the house for an hour or two, once or twice a week. These earnings gave them incentive to work and taught them the value of labor and monetary wages. Some of the paid jobs that went beyond their usual daily duties were organizing cupboards, deep-cleaning closets, and mopping the kitchen floor.

If you want **CHILDREN** to keep *their feet on the* GROUND, *put some* responsibility on their SHOULDERS

Abigail Van Buren

Children should begin doing small jobs as soon as they are old enough to understand your requests, such as picking up toys, carrying folded clothes to their bedroom, carrying a loaf of bread from the car into the house, or standing on a stool near a table beside you to pour ingredients into a bowl when cooking or baking. If a new baby is in the house, a toddler can give a doll a bath, at the same time you bathe the infant. A small child can bring a clean diaper when you're changing the baby. They can also put soap in the washer or clothes in the dryer. They can help plant a seed or weed the garden.

Involve the child in your daily duties to make them feel useful and to learn the value of work at an early age. Small accomplishments will help a child's confidence grow and encourage him or her to work, especially when followed by praise, hugs, kisses, a pat on the back, a cheer, a hoot, a holler, or a happy dance. Words of affirmation such as, "You did a good job!" or "You're such a good helper!" will motivate a child to work. You can also tuck a note of encouragement, praise, or a few kind words in your older children's lunch boxes or on their dressers. These words of acceptance, affirmation, and praise are like precious jewels deposited in their hearts to increase their sense of self-worth.

EXPERIMENT AND INVENT

When we fulfill every whim that children often want, or every little need that they can often do for themselves, we are denying them the opportunity to grow into resourceful adults. Having a genuine need or desire stimulates the imagination and fuels ingenuity to find a solution. Necessity forces the mind to search for and find answers. A child may see a need, discover a solution, and become an inventor, engineer, or pioneer. If you think your child is too young to invent, see how the following children created prototypes of things that we use today.

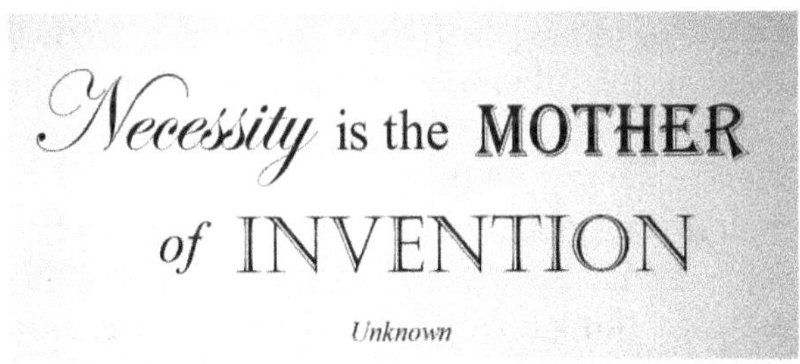

Henry Ford began taking watches apart, putting them back together, and then repairing broken ones before he was even a teenager. He made his own makeshift tools from objects around the house. He became a self-taught machinist and then began working as an apprentice in a machine shop in his early teens. A few years later, his diligence, experience, and ingenuity helped him create the moving assembly line that made cars more affordable for the masses.

Thomas Edison was seven years-old when he was labeled retarded and unable to learn by his primary grade teacher, so Nancy Edison began teaching her son at home. She encouraged him to read, and Thomas devoured books by the dozens. A few years later, he created a chemistry lab in the family's basement to use for experiments. Thomas also began working for the railroad when he was twelve years-old, selling food, and his own published newspapers to passengers. Thomas made friends with the telegraph operators on the railway stops, where he acquired knowledge about the telegraph, all before he was sixteen years old.. He later went on to patent over 1,000 inventions during his lifetime.

Orville and Wilber Wright's mother influenced her sons by encouraging them to read and build, which fueled their curiosity and creativity. She was also a role model because of her mechanical abilities, making toys for the boys and appliances for her home. The Wright Brothers read books from their vast home library, which included books on ornithology. No doubt that their study and knowledge of birds played an important part in their quest to finding a way for man to fly.

These great inventors all had mothers or fathers who allowed them to take things apart and put them back together, tinker with ideas and thingamajigs, build crazy contraptions, and experiment with gizmos and gadgets that were unheard of during their lifetimes. All the while instilling internal values and solidifying high standards to help them become some of the greatest inventors of all time.

Lesser known young inventors include Joseph-Armand Bombardier, a 15 year old who in 1922 put his dad's Model-T onto a sled, and the concept of the snowmobile was born. There's George Nissen, a 16-year-old high school gymnast who in 1930 invented the trampoline. We also have Philo Farnsworth, the 14-year-old boy, who in 1920 conceived of the television. Seven years later he and his business partner transmitted the first-ever images onto the screen.

Teenagers have also invented Braille (15 years-old), Popsicles (11 years-old), earmuffs (15 years-old), and a promising test for pancreatic cancer (15 years-old). On a more current note, a 12 year-old boy has invented a Braille printer made out of Lego blocks!

The American psychologist, Abraham Maslow, said that almost all creativity involves purposeful play. Listen to your children's dreams. Have faith in their abilities. Then give them free rein to experiment with their "crazy" ideas. If you see unusual gifts or talents in your children, nurture and encourage their natural abilities rather than steer them down the well-trodden path of conformity.

GET A JOB AND GET PAID

Work can be "fun" if you find a job that you enjoy and it makes you feel good inside. Knowing that your contribution in the workforce is making a difference in lives can also make the job a fulfilling endeavor. Even if the work is not very enjoyable, a feeling of accomplishment and pride can be gained, knowing that you're making your own way in the world, or that you are helping to provide for someone else's needs besides your own.

It's not what you've GOT,
it's *how* you **USE IT.**
success is a matter of ATTITUDE.

If your children are over fourteen years-old they are able to get a part-time job, but they may need working papers. Check with the Department of Labor in your state (www.dol.gov/dol/location.htm) to find a location where they can apply for the necessary documents. School guidance counselors can help facilitate this process as well.

When seeking employment, children should be courteous and confident when asking friends or neighbors for a job and when stating their hourly fee. Doing a job well, possibly hearing praise, and getting paid for their work will increase their confidence and teach them skills that will help them later in life. Responsibility and accountability which are fueled by work help build the character traits of dependability and loyalty. Small jobs done well at an early age are stepping stones that lead to a successful future in the workforce.

The child may also develop a sense of camaraderie when working side-by-side with other people. This teamwork often creates a bond that can develop into a friendship that may last a lifetime.

Fourteen to Sixteen Years-Old

Children in their early teens can do quite a few things to make extra money. Some of these jobs were mentioned in the volunteer section. The difference between that list and this one is that the previous list was meant for those who were unable to do for themselves or who may be struggling to make ends meet. This list is for customers who are able to do for themselves, but may not have time to accomplish these jobs because of their own work schedule.

- Offer to mow a lawn.
- Offer to shovel snow.
- Offer to wash windows.
- Offer to wash and wax cars.
- Offer to pull weeds from a flower bed.
- Apply for a job tying grapes in the spring.
- Apply for a job picking fruits or vegetables.
- Apply for a job doing housecleaning at www.care.com.
- Apply for a job running errands at www.care.com.
- Make beautiful or useful crafts and sell them. Find ideas on Pinterest.
- Apply for a job cleaning or painting for landlords who own rental properties.
- If you have the means and space to do so, plant a small garden and then sell cut flowers, tomatoes, green beans, peppers, or lettuce at a roadside stand.
- If you live outside the city limits and you have the means to do so, buy and raise chickens and then sell

the eggs. Find out how at www.almanac.com / Raising Chickens 101.

- Make hula hoops by following a YouTube tutorial and then sell them for a profit. One roll of ¾" irrigation tubing will make about ten hoops. After buying couplers and colored electrical, floral, or duct tape to decorate them, you will need a blow-dryer and a hacksaw (for an adult to cut the tubing). The total cost of supplies is approximately $50. Even if each hoop is sold for a mere $10 (or up to $20), you will make a $50 (to $150) profit.

Sixteen to Eighteen Years-Old

When a child is old enough to own a cell phone (that has a monthly fee) or to drive a car (that will raise your insurance premiums), they are old enough to get a part-time job to cover the cost of these *privileges*. This is not being mean to them. It is helping them learn how to generate an income and survive on their own in life.

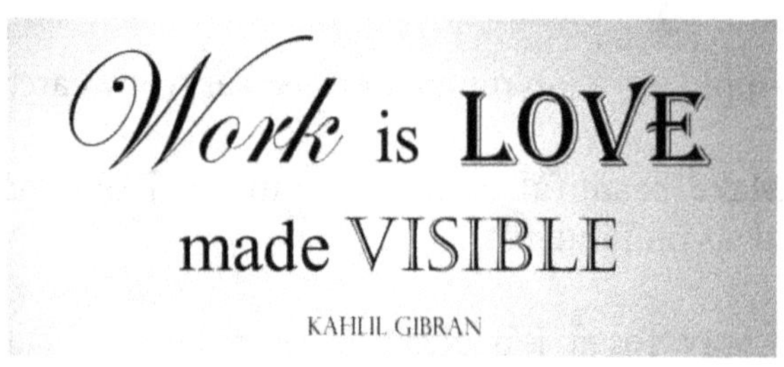

In addition to the suggestions above, older teens can apply for some of the following jobs. If they choose to become self-employed, they can make business cards to offer their services and expected wages, by printing them out on the computer or by ordering them at Vistaprint.com or 123Print.com. Look online for discount codes or free shipping codes toward these printing services.

Help your child open a savings or checking account. A sixteen year old can usually open an account with parental consent and a signature. A bank account not only prepares them for adulthood, but it also gives them a feeling of responsibility and builds self-esteem. They can also fill out a resume and post their references and availability of services at www.care.com or make flyers and post them at business entrances (with permission, of course).

- Factory worker.
- Cashier in a store.
- Server at a restaurant.
- Newspaper deliveries.
- Seasonal work on a farm.
- Pump fuel at a gas station.
- Seasonal work in a department store.
- Seasonal work at a concession stand.
- Sandwich maker at a deli or sub shop.
- Bus tables or wash dishes in a restaurant.
- Painting stairs, walls, porches, barns, fences.
- Restock grocery or department store shelves.
- Become a lifeguard through your local Red Cross.

- Become a pet-sitter or dog walker through www.care.com.

- Maintain someone's car for them (rotate tires, check fluids, change the oil).

- Become a babysitter through www.care.com. Take a class in child care and first aid through the Red Cross.

- Open a PayPal account and sell your stuff on eBay (check out other sellers' pages to learn how to write exciting descriptions of your merchandise. Scour household sales and buy old toys, vintage clothes, and other interesting items to sell).

- Write, edit, and create a book and cover and then submit your poems, stories, or non-fiction articles to Amazon's KDP program, Barnes & Noble's Nook Press program, and Smashwords multi-distribution site for publication and distribution. Research blogs about book marketing and then promote your work and get paid for it.

Children learn to manage money by earning an income and being allowed to pay their way for non-essentials. This cash becomes their spending money and savings so they are not dependent on you for every dollar they desire. Children gain confidence when they discover the joy in a job well done, and the monetary reward of hard work. Shielding a child from work is not a form of protection. On the contrary, it stunts their physical, mental, emotional, and social growth. Work is indeed love made visible.

BE A GOOD-DEED-DOER

When the world famous comedienne, Lucille Ball, was fourteen years-old and living in Celeron, New York, she went to a dance wearing a beautiful taffeta dress trimmed with fur that her mother had sewn. A less fortunate girl admired the elegant dress and Lucy took note. The next day, Lucy took the expensive dress and gave it to the girl without any strings attached. [19] This generous attitude most likely contributed to Lucille Ball's successful career in future years.

> Ten rules for getting rid of the BLUES. Go out and do something for someone else. REPEAT NINE TIMES.

A surefire way to be happy is to make someone else happy. When you bring joy into a person's life, you also receive joy into your life too. Voilà! Helping others is one of the best ways to help yourself!

What you give out is what you get back. It works just like a boomerang as spiritual and natural laws kick into effect. Corn stalks grow when a kernel of corn is buried in the ground. Tomatoes grow when tomato seeds are sown in the soil. In every planting situation, you must let something go to get something back. You never reap corn by *holding onto* seeds, and you never reap corn by planting petunia seeds. You always get back exactly what you plant.

Not only that but when you plant one seed, that one seed produces *many* more seeds when the fruit is ripe. Whatever you give out *always* produces more of its kind *in abundance*. Therefore, it logically stands to reason that whatever you want to come back to you, you must give that thing away. The Bible verse that says, *Give and it shall be given unto you*, applies to *everything.* Whatever you give will come back to you whether it's *good or bad.*

If you want to grow love, you must give love. If you want to grow joy, you must plant gratitude in every situation. If you hope to gather many friends, you must sow seeds of kindness to *every person you meet.* People never reap peace by sowing discord, and they never grow love by sowing mean seeds, because the natural and spiritual laws must return that which was planted, which in these cases are strife and loneliness.

Therefore, plant only good seeds that will produce a harvest of good things. Scatter more and you will gather more, and gain a bumper crop of blessings. Stingy giving produces limited living. Generous giving produces abundant living, so scatter liberally.

When you do good deeds, you're planting good seeds that will bring joy and purpose to your life and benefits to the recipients. The following examples of meaningful deeds can be done on a regular basis, or on occasion. Invite a friend to join you in this fun and fulfilling endeavor, and you will double your pleasure by forming a closer relationship with them in the process too.

This list is similar to the previous section on volunteering your services, but it is slightly different. Doing good deeds are more assertive than volunteer work. You are not asking permission to do these things like a volunteer does. You are taking it upon yourself to do something good, or kind, or helpful for someone else, by simply taking action.

Many of these deeds need money to carry through, so what can you do? One way to come up with the cash is by taking ten percent of your earnings and using it to help someone else. If that is not possible, give what you can to those who are less fortunate than you, no matter what the amount.

The joy and fulfillment that you receive will be worth the expense. Go out of your way to make someone's life better and always try to be generous. When you add a ray of sunshine to someone else's life, you can't help but brighten your own life too. Here are a few suggestions to get you started.

- Feed a quarter to an expired parking meter.
- Give someone a Mason jar full of wildflowers.
- Give carnations to people outside a grocery store.
- Carry groceries to an elderly woman's car or her front door.
- Donate new or used books to the comfort room in a cancer hospital.
- Make or bake a healthy meal and take it to someone who lives alone.
- Give your parents a hug and thank them for all they've done for you.
- Hold the door open for the person behind you and let them go in first.
- Donate a gently-used coat or a pair of boots or shoes to a needy person.
- Pick up litter in your neighborhood then recycle it or throw it in the trash.

- Download an audio-book and gift it to someone who is visually impaired.
- Organize a fundraiser to bring an inspirational guest speaker to your school.
- Buy a grocery store gift card or a bag of groceries and give it to a needy family.
- Leave a box of small Christmas gifts at a needy family's door during the holidays.
- Donate canned or dry goods to a women's shelter, a soup kitchen, or a food pantry.
- Make copies of inspirational quotes and then put them under car windshield wipers.
- Leave a box of groceries at a needy person's door without them finding out who left it.
- Hand out cold bottles of water to runners, walkers, bikers, or a road crew on a hot day.
- Plant spices like parsley, basil, or cilantro in small terracotta pots and then give them away.
- Pass out glow sticks from the Dollar Store to kids watching fireworks on the Fourth of July.
- Participate in the national "Make a Difference Day," and send your story to the press at makeadifferenceday.com

- Pass out carnations to teachers, waitresses, cashiers, or sales staff to show your appreciation for the work that they do.

- Leave a Post-it note on someone's car window that says, *You are important! Smile!* or *Have a great day!* (Then add a smiley face.)

- Get a group of friends together and start a beautification project in your community. Plant flowers, trees, or shrubs in a barren area.

- Get a group of kids together, make a few dozen healthy sandwiches, and then pass them out, along with bottles of water to homeless people.

- Look for bottles and cans while out walking and then take them to the recycle station. Use the money to buy any of the "good-deed" items mentioned in this section.

- Assist anyone who seems to be struggling. Carry someone's packages for them. Help an elderly or disabled person across the street. Offer your seat if someone is standing.

- Befriend a lonely classmate at school. Invite him or her to sit with you during lunch. Offer to walk him or her home from school. Invite him or her to a kid-friendly movie and then pay for the theater ticket.

- Send a note of encouragement to someone who is having a difficult time. Slip a few dollars in an envelope or a stick of sugarless gum, and then write something like, "Just a little note to say, you are in my thoughts (prayers) today."

- Sweep floors, do dishes, clean bathrooms, and change sheets for someone who is ill or caring for someone who is ill.

- Prepare a nutritious meal complete with side dishes and bread, and then take it to someone who is struggling physically or financially.

- Get a group of kids together and do a beach sweep or a street cleanup in your city. Bring gloves, rakes, brooms, shovels, and trash bags. Call the newspaper to cover the event and it may encourage others to do similar projects.

- Clean your room from top to bottom and then donate gently used clothes, toys, games, or anything else that you don't use anymore, to needy children or to a charity such as a Thrift Store or to a church that sends goods to impoverished countries.

- Send hand-written notes or homemade cards of appreciation to teachers, teachers' aids, librarians, principals, policemen, or firemen. Thank them for their service, time and dedication, then send the letter snail mail, slip it under their door, or deliver it in person.

- Recruit a friend to help you wash car windshields in a parking lot. Gather up a squeegee and a bucket of window cleaner and then have fun for one hour. Leave a cheery note when you're finished, such as "A bit of sparkle to brighten your day." (Add a smiley face).

- Take a gift basket full of goodies to a child who is ill or going through a difficult time. Fill it with things like a DVD, magazines, coloring books, crayons, a small flashlight, puzzles, activity books, lip balm, glow-sticks, nightlights, or a plastic cup with a character on it.

- Create a care-kit for a homeless person or a struggling college student. Buy a plastic shoebox-sized container with a lid and then add things like razors, a comb, shampoo, soap, hand-sanitizer, a toothbrush, toothpaste, deodorant, Band-Aids, lip balm, socks, disposable wipes, easy-open cans of tuna, juice boxes, a plastic poncho, a gift card for a haircut, a small Bible, or any other useful items.

- Create a team that will help you connect with grocery stores or restaurants to see what they dispose of (in order to make room for fresher baked goods, produce, and other foods). Many restaurants throw away take-out orders that are not picked up. Many grocery stores toss out perfectly good food in order to make room for new shipments. Approach the managers and ask if you can collect and distribute this food to the homeless. Be sure to find out if this is legal in your county or state.

- Recruit friends to host a benefit for someone who has a great financial need. Set up an event like a carnival with games and prizes to raise money for a worthy cause. Make up baskets for a Chinese auction. Paint life-sized cartoon pictures of people on cardboard refrigerator boxes and then cut holes in them for the faces. Approach local businesses for donations, contributions, or other means of support. Contact managers of grocery stores, department stores, restaurants, and other places of service to see if they will donate food, merchandise, a hall with a kitchen area, or their services via gift certificates to your cause.

One kind act a day has a way of transforming, not only the life of the person receiving the good deed, but also the life of the doer of the good deed. Small acts of kindness and service can change a situation, almost like magic. But it's not magic. It's a spiritual law that goes into effect once you take the first step. Even *giving* words of praise or encouragement to someone, especially someone who feels downtrodden, will not only lift his or her spirits, but also yours as well. Helping someone who has a need can be a powerful antidote for the blues. Giving someone a compliment also has a way of making *you* feel better too, so it's a win-win situation.

KNOW THYSELF

Shakespeare said in one of his plays, "To thine own self be true." I interpret this quote as one that means, don't forfeit your values to please other people. Don't lower your standards to win friends, or run races with meaningless ends. Being true to yourself is also *being yourself*, not an imitation of someone else. It's being loyal to God and to love and to doing what's right, all of which work on your behalf to garner your highest good. When you are true to yourself, you will also be less likely swayed by harmful influences, or negative expectations from other people.

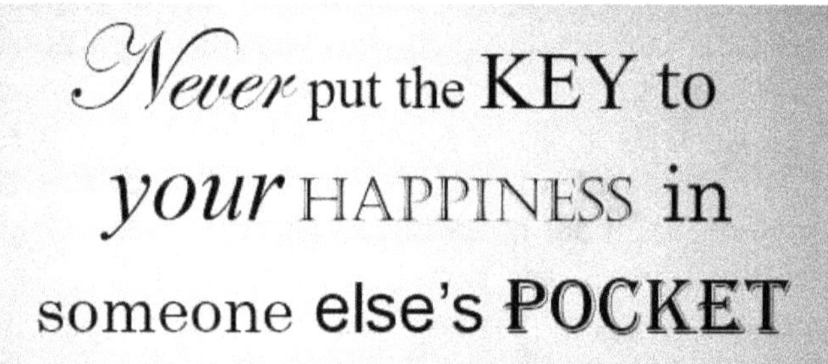

This section is about direction and discerning the best course for your life. Having a clear purpose or Truth keeps a person from getting lost or meandering all over the place. It also prevents a person on the right path from straying down rabbit-trails. It also gives a person the strength and determination to continue going forward when the road is rocky or the sky is stormy. But first, you must know where you are, before you can get where you want to go.

Where are you?

If you look at a map, you tell yourself, "I am here, but I want to go there" (where "X" marks the spot on the map). A few ways to determine where you are is to take inventory of your life. This written reflection is similar to looking in a mirror to fix your hair, wash your face, or make other external adjustments.

A few questions to begin this inward reflection may be: *Who am I? Why am I here? What is my ultimate purpose in life?* Another way to jump-start this effort is to make a list of 25 things that you appreciate or 25 things that make you happy. Making this list will reveal your priorities.

Unload the Trunk

Before you venture out on a trip, you must clear the trunk before loading the luggage. Creative journaling or writing poetry, songs, or short stories may help you express yourself and provide a release for emotions that are difficult to say aloud.

Journaling can also be a form of immortality. Once you write down your life stories, values, ideas, and beliefs, you can leave a legacy for future generations. Other formats besides a notebook can provide more privacy such as a locked Word file, or an ongoing email draft to your own email address. There are also many free and paid apps available that serve this purpose.

This private freedom of expression is often therapeutic. When you write down your ideas, feelings and experiences, the process may also help organize your thoughts and prioritize your life. The questions in the "Swimming in the Deep" section may also be a springboard that leads to self-discovery.

Where do you want to go?

In the game of billiards, the winner is the one who *calls the shot* and hits the ball in the *specified pocket.* Setting goals work in a similar way. One of the greatest secrets to reaching goals is to write them down in vivid detail rather than sweeping generalizations.

For example, if I asked my neighbor to purchase some meat for me at the grocery store, she wouldn't know what to buy, because the request is too general. If I asked her to buy two pounds of meat that would still be too vague. If I said I wanted chicken or chicken breasts that would be better, but still not specific enough. To be very precise, I would say two pounds of boneless, skinless chicken breasts. I could even add a brand name to make it more specific. The point is that your goals should be just as detailed and clear, so that when you write your list, you will know exactly what you're aiming for on the target.

I learned this lesson during my senior year of high school while daydreaming during class. I flipped to the back of my marble notebook and wrote down a list of things that I wanted to buy and things that I wanted to do in the future, even though I had no job or means to reach these goals. I listed items like a denim jacket, my own apartment, and four vacation destinations among other things. Within six months, I had all of the tangible items on my list, and within three years I traveled to the four places I'd listed. I learned a very important lesson that day. One that I've used ever since with great success.

After you write down your short and long term goals, it is important to review and revise the list on a regular basis. It is also important to believe that the attainment of your specific dreams is possible. Once you do this, you can go even further into the future and determine your priorities and goals from a deathbed perspective. This may sound a bit morbid, but if you keep this perspective in mind, your priorities naturally fall into place. This eternal outlook is similar to shaking sand and gravel in a sifter. The insignificant falls away and leaves behind the gold.

So grab a notebook and a pen and begin listing your goals in various categories. Many people begin with careers, vacations, or material things at the top of their lists, but think of ways to improve your health, education, and relationships too. Taking personal inventory and writing down your goals should be a lifelong habit. Many things will hinder your progress and you may not hit the bull's eye each time, but if you aim for the center and miss, you still should hit the target. Either way, your life will be better than if you didn't take the shot at all.

DISPENSE YOUR AFFECTION

One of the questions I asked in the "Deepen Your Relationships" section was, *If you were going to lose one of your senses, and you had the ability to choose which one, what would it be?* Most people cannot fathom life without the gift of sight, and on first impulse, that was my choice, because I love to see vibrant colors, lights, and beautiful sights, and because life in general would be difficult without the ability to see.

Yet, there is one sense that would make life almost unbearable if it was gone, and that is the sense of touch. You might think it would be great not to feel any pain, but even that has drawbacks. History has shown that lepers felt no pain, and as a result, they lost body parts from burns and cuts and excessive pressure, among other things. Those who lost their sense of touch and the ability to feel, never knew there was a problem until it was too late.

To feel no pain also means to feel no pleasure. Without the sense of touch, there would be no sensory awareness of affection or physical intimacy. Studies have shown that babies in orphanages who were not held, cuddled, rocked, and stroked died for no apparent reason other than they simply failed to thrive, due to lack of touch.

Most young children are naturally affectionate and enjoy lots of hugs, kisses, snuggles, and cuddles. Many teens are not so open to such loving gestures. Older children may push you away, because they feel they're too old for this type of affection. But they also need loving touch to thrive in life and stay close to you. It may also shield them from the lure of seeking premature or misguided affection from their friends.

So how do you fill this important need if they don't want hugs and kisses anymore? Offer to braid or brush your daughter's hair while watching a movie together. Playfully tickle her back *in passing,* or offer to paint her fingernails. Quickly rub your son's shoulders or back *in passing*. Sneak in a quick side hug when standing next to him. Touch your hand on his or her shoulder when you walk past them. Playfully insist that *you* need a hug in exchange for the car keys. Organize a game of touch football with family members. Most of these demonstrative deeds must be done quickly. Get in-and-out like lightning. Act as though it's not a big deal, even though it is a huge deal.

Touch is like glue. It bonds people together. Keep your children close to you by giving them time and attention, along with playful and loving affection.

***

Thank you for reading *I'm Hungry! I'm Bored!* I hope that you enjoyed it. If you found this book helpful, please consider posting an online review so others may benefit too.

Much love and many blessings from me to you.

Carol McCormick

KUDOS

I would like to thank my pre-publication readers and editors for their sharp eyes and fabulous input: Donna Berg, Kris Dziduch, Dan George, Tracy McCormick, Heidi Payne, and Sharon Perdue. You have all been amazing!

If you do find errors in this book, dear reader, please contact me so I can make the necessary corrections. I take full responsibility for them after adding last minute tweaks to the manuscript, *after* the editors had completed their work. My email address is cjmccor2002@hotmail.com. Thank you.

I would also like to thank Amy Estep for her wonderful photography skills, and Gavin Estep, Abagail, Benjamin, Nicholas, and Sophie Davis for their beautiful smiling faces.

I would also like to thank Kempo Karate, Crino Music, and the Dunkirk Free Library for the use of their facilities for the photo sessions.

Without you all, this book would not be what it is today! Thank you! Thank you! Thank you!

ENDNOTES

[1] Appleton High School Study: www.thewholeplate.yihs.net/wp-content/uploads/2010/02/Appleton-school-food-study.pdf

[2] Thirty Percent of the World is Overweight: www.nbcnews.com/health/diet-fitness/whole-world-getting-fatter-new-survey-finds-n115811

[3] Jared's Weight Loss Journey via Subway: www.subway.com/subwayroot/freshbuzz/Jared/default.aspx

[4] Vitamin B6 / ADHD: www.ncbi.nlm.nih.gov/pubmed/16846100

[5] Magnesium / ADD and ADHD: www.ncbi.nlm.nih.gov/pubmed/16846100

[6] Iron / ADHD: www.ncbi.nlm.nih.gov/pubmed/18054688

[7] Zinc / ADHD: www.ncbi.nlm.nih.gov/pubmed/21309695

[8] Omega-3's Many Benefits: nccam.nih.gov/health/tips/omega

[9] Pamela Peeke, MD, MPH, FACP, "Food and Addiction: The Dopamine Made Me Do It," *IDEA Fitness Journal for ACE certified professionals,* October 2012: www.drpeeke.com/data/images/food_addition_october_2012_with_cover.pdf

[10] Jack LaLanne, "God Father of Fitness": www.jacklalanne.com/jacks-adventures/king-of-fitness.php

[11] Queen Elizabeth's Black Teeth: www.historyonthenet.com/tudors/elizabeth_portrait_of_a_queen.htm

[12] Non-alcoholic fatty liver: www.ncbi.nlm.nih.gov/pmc/articles/PMC3735407/

[13] Cartwright, Martina M., PhD, RD, “The Stimulating Truth about Energy Drinks,” *IDEA Fitness Journal for ACE certified professionals,* June 2013.www.ideafit.com/fitness-library/the-stimulating-truth-about-energy-drinks

[14] National Center for Biotechnology Information on Caffeine: www.ncbi.nlm.nih.gov/pmc/articles/PMC3065144/

[15] Benefits of Honey: www.smithsonianmag.com/science-nature/the-science-behind-honeys-eternal-shelf-life-1218690/

[16] The Story of my Life by Helen Keller. Letters written by Annie Sullivan: www.afb.org/mylife/book.asp?ch=p3ch3

[17] Pamela Peeke, MD, MPH, FACP, “Food and Addiction: The Dopamine Made Me Do It,” *IDEA* October 2012: www.drpeeke.com/data/images/food_addition_october_2012_with_cover.pdf

[18] Keep it Natural www.psychologytoday.com/blog/your-neurochemical-self/201212/five-ways-boost-your-natural-happy-chemicals

[19] Ball, Lucille, *Love Lucy*, G.P. Putnam’s Sons, New York, 1996

RESOURCES

www.eatright.org

www.medlineplus.gov

www.letsmove.gov

www.wholegrainscouncil.org

www.choosemyplate.gov

www.fda.gov/Food U. S. Food & Drug Administration

www.health.gov/dietaryguidelines

www.cancer.gov/cancertopics/factsheet/Risk/artificial-sweeteners

www.cdc.gov Centers for Disease Control and Prevention/nutrition

www.cnpp.usda.gov: Center for Nutrition Policy and Promotion / United States Department of Agriculture

www.fooducate.com Free app scans a product's barcode and scores its nutritional value

www.healthpartners.com/yumpower Ideas and tips for kid's nutrition

www.healthydiningfinder.com Healthy Dining Finder to find healthy food choices offered at area restaurants

Find the best times for sun exposure and Vitamin D absorption with this free app: www.dminder.ontometrics.com

www.hhs.gov Department of Health and Human Services

www.myfitnesspal.com: Free calorie and nutrition app

www.supertracker.usda.gov/ Free personalized nutrition and physical activity plan, track your progress, and get health related tips and support

www.usda.gov United Stated Department of Agriculture

www.who.int/topics/obesity/en/ World Health Organization

Talk to Me! Listen to Me!

Keys to Improve Communication and Questions to Deepen Relationships

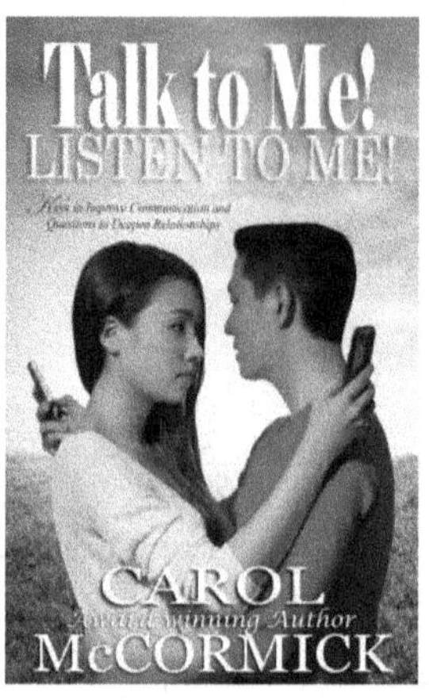

When thoughts and feelings are expressed during deep levels of communication, true intimacy is established and attachments are formed that are fairly unbreakable. Today, we see more and more people interacting electronically rather than enjoying face-to-face or side-by-side conversations. As a result, rather than feeling more connected, people often feel more disconnected than ever. *Talk to Me! Listen to Me!* is a tool to help turn things around with its many suggestions and 150 questions.

"The majority of people's problems are caused by the fact that they are disconnected with the rest of creation." C.S. Lewis

Available at online bookstores
carolmccormick.com

The Missing Piece

Award-winning Inspirational Love Story

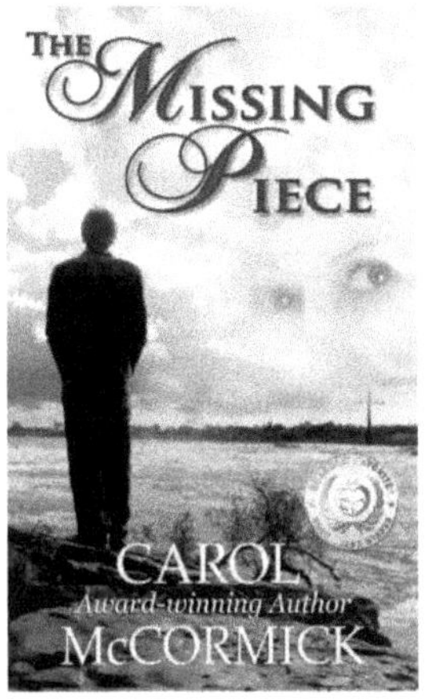

"Fresh dialogue, realistic characters, a powerful message. McCormick does a great job creating her characters and portraying the struggles they endure," The Romance Readers Connection

How does a man pick up the pieces when his world crashes around him? Misplaced priorities shattered his marriage. Problems almost crushed him. Love motivated him to mend the damage, once he found all the pieces.

Available at online bookstores and Audible.com
carolmccormick.com

Your Special Gift
A Preteen Primer to the Facts of Life

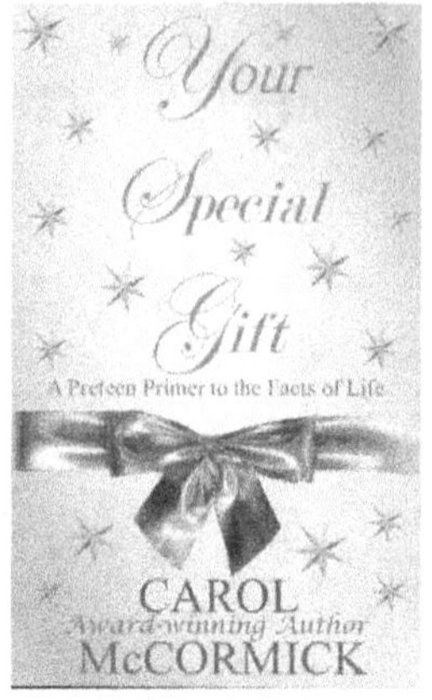

"*Your Special Gift* is a wonderful booklet for parents to share with their adolescent children!" Marjorie Holmes, bestselling author

The simplicity of the gift, lock, and key analogy opens the door of communication between adult and child in an effective straightforward, and yet sensitive way, so that any question concerning sex can be answered by using this method. Well-suited for 8-to-12 year-old children.

If you don't tell them, someone else will.

Available at online bookstores and audible.com
carolmccormick.com

Window Pains

Modeling Positive Behaviors

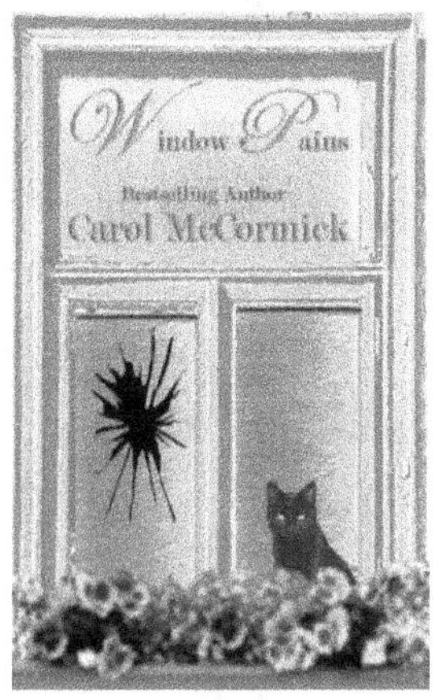

Window Pains is a short story that was originally published in *WINNER*, a scholastic magazine endorsed by a former president and two former first ladies. The aim of the periodical was to teach children preventative measures and to instill positive behaviors that contribute to success in life.

Window Pains briefly deals with peer pressure and restitution. Discussion questions are included. Ideal for 7-to-12 year-old children.

Available at online bookstores and audible.com
carolmccormick.com

www.ingramcontent.com/pod-product-compliance
Lightning Source LLC
Chambersburg PA
CBHW072122270326
41931CB00010B/1640

* 9 7 8 0 9 6 7 5 3 6 8 2 8 *